Stretching

for Flexibility and Health

Francine St. George

THE CROSSING PRESS
FREEDOM, CALIFORNIA

For information on bulk purchases or group discounts for this and other
Crossing Press titles, please contact our Special Sales Manager at 800-777-1048.

Visit our Website on the Internet at: www.crossingpress.com

Library of Congress Cataloging-in-Publication Data
St. George, Francine.
Stretching for flexibility & health / Francine St. George.
p. cm.
Includes index.
ISBN 0-89594-882-6 (paper)
1. Stretching exercises. 2. Muscle strength. I. Title.
RA781.63.S7 1997
613.7'1--dc21   97-24476
                                                                          CIP

All the exercises in this book should be performed with care, and are under-
taken at the reader's sole discretion and risk.

Acknowledgments

My first thanks must go to the readers of *The Muscle Fitness Book*. Their suggestions have resulted in the many new exercises and revised text of *Stretching for Flexibility and Health*. Thanks also to my patients, as their many questions have helped me to determine much of the content of the book.

I thank my clinic colleagues for permitting me time to complete the book. In particular, I would like to thank Heather Bastert for her typing expertise and valuable feedback on the manuscript.

A special thanks to Josie Howlett for her artwork; to Jonathan Chester for his photography; to George Sirett for his design; to my publisher Kirsty Melville for her guidance with the direction of the book; and to my editor Elizabeth Neate for her patience and skill at all stages of the publishing process.

Contents

Foreword

Most of us accept that getting fit involves doing some form of aerobic exercise, but how many of us realize the important part that stretching and strengthening exercises have to play in a fitness regime? In her physical therapy clinic Francine St. George has been using these exercises for many years as an integral part of her treatment program for sportspeople and those in chronic pain.

As an elite athlete and now as a busy consultant I have needed to see a physical therapist at various times. I have consulted Francine over the last ten years and I have always found her recommended exercises beneficial in maintaining flexibility, strength and overall fitness. In fact, whenever life becomes so busy that I neglect these exercises, I find that my general fitness level drops.

In this book, Francine has drawn on her considerable experience and research to present 130 of the most effective exercises, as well as providing a thorough account of muscle fitness in general. She has also answered the need for a book that combines both muscle and heart/lung fitness by showing how to incorporate the stretching and strengthening exercises into an overall fitness regime.

Most importantly, Francine has written a book that can be used by everyone — from elite athletes to the beginner starting a fitness program. I look forward to it being in my own library for my personal use, and I have no hesitation in recommending it as a valuable contribution to the health and fitness area.

Yours in Sport

Dawn Fraser

Dawn Fraser

Introduction

The excuse "I am too busy to find time to exercise" is becoming all too common. The combination of sedentary daily work and hectic schedules means that keeping fit is indeed a challenge.

In my physicaltherapy clinic I see patients with a wide range of muscle and joint problems, and I find it intriguing that so many have injured themselves at their busiest times, when exercise has been *accidentally* neglected for weeks, months, or even years. As a adjunct to treatment, I usually prescribe stretching and strengthening exercises. While my patients are recovering, they are very committed to their exercises — they will do anything to help alleviate their pain. However, as their pain goes, so does their regular exercise regime. Sadly, a cycle begins, and a few months later they are back in my clinic, telling me the same story of neck or back pain, or wherever it is that stress has made them vulnerable. Can you relate to this cycle of pain and lack of exercise? It is a common scenario encountered within any treatment clinic.

Ironically, with athletes — that is, people who exercise regularly, either socially or competitively — the opposite syndrome occurs. They may feel a slight pain, for instance, while going for their regular jog, but they feel that if they ignore it, it will go away. Ever fearful that their physical therapist will say "rest", they continue to jog until pain forces them to stop. The physical therapist's role is now difficult: not only does it involve treating the original painful area, but it also involves clearing the multiple other complaints developed in the attempt to keep exercising. Rest is inevitable at this stage, yet if attention had been sought sooner, the time out of the activity could have been greatly reduced.

Both these situations — underexercising and overexercising — are familiar to any health practitioner. Yet with a little knowledge of some basic rules about body fitness, the repetitive cycle of pain and injury due to lack of fitness or too much exercise can be avoided. The advances in sports science in the 1980s, particularly in the areas of health and fitness and the athlete, have meant that the importance of maintaining a regular fitness program, but not doing too much, is now accepted categorically. A fit body can reduce your risk of injury and of cardiovascular disease, both so prevalent in our society.

However, when my patients ask me where they can find the information on exercise-related questions, or how they can remember exercises when they are not needing treatment, I have found the existing books either too technical or too simple. *Stretching for Flexibility and Health* was written to meet this need.

Based on the popular *Muscle Fitness Book*, it provides information that is less technical and more suitable for readers at all levels of fitness. It offers many new exercises that I have found to be excellent for improving general flexibility, and, in clinical practice, for treating patients with recurrent neck or back pain. Though initially you may find them challenging, after persevering with appropriately selected exercises, you will note a dramatic improvement in your posture and, furthermore, you will feel good!

Stretching for Flexibility and Health outlines the basics about getting fit and staying fit in ten easy-to-follow stages. If you are wishing to start an exercise or a fitness program, the information and exercises within will make the task of getting started and maintaining a regular routine easy and fun. If you are currently engaged in regular exercise or involved in a specific sport, this book will help you to reduce your risk of injury. Health professionals, personal trainers and gymnasium personnel will also find the book useful when prescribing exercise programs.

The first two chapters focus on understanding the body and clarifying the facts on muscles. Particular emphasis is on the musculoskeletal and cardiovascular systems, the most important systems for muscle fitness. The muscles relevant to the exercises that are shown later are illustrated and briefly discussed.

Chapter 3 reviews the answers to the questions regarding muscles that I am often asked in my clinical practice, while Chapters 4 and 5 identify the issues you will need to be aware of when you are starting a fitness program and/or preparing and training for sport — these chapters are important to review no matter what your level of fitness.

Probably one of the most important aspects of muscle fitness is stretching. Chapter 6 reviews why it is important to stretch, both daily to improve general flexibility, and before and after sporting activity to avoid injury. Chapter 7 then covers stretching and strengthening exercises for the entire body, commencing with the neck and shoulders, progressing to the trunk and abdomen, and then to the hips and lower limbs. Potentially dangerous exercises are also shown, along with safe alternatives.

Chapter 8 provides daily flexibility and strengthening regimes; these should be done in conjunction with aerobic exercise for overall muscle fitness. Chapter 9 outlines exercises for specific groups. General stretches suitable prior to and at the completion of your sporting activity are included here. You will need to choose the exercises that are appropriate to your sport.

These should only take a few minutes to do prior to your sport, but should be combined with a regular stretching regime to work on overall body flexibility, as most sports do not use all muscles in the body evenly. Exercises to avoid back pain or to prevent a recurrence of a back complaint are also provided in this chapter.

Chapter 10 provides the basics on how to take care of your muscles if you do sustain an injury, and, of course, how to avoid one.

With regular stretching, you will be surprised at how quickly your overall flexibility and muscle tone will improve. You will also feel more relaxed in your muscles generally and will be able to avoid the pain and injury cycle. Though it is a challenge, you *can* fit a daily fitness regime into a seemingly impossible schedule. I know that I wouldn't be able to survive my work as physical therapist, lecturer, and researcher, among my other roles, without my daily exercise and stretching. By doing a different form of exercise each day and varying my fitness regime, I have made it possible.

So, good luck with keeping fit, enjoy the prereading and always have fun!

How to Use This Book

To gain the most from this book, read through the first few chapters before going to the exercises. This will make keeping fit more fun, as well as giving you a better understanding of the reasons for doing so.

Following the daily routines is a simple way for you to achieve muscle fitness, but they should be combined with regular aerobic activity for overall muscle and heart/lung fitness. As an alternative to following the daily routines, you may wish to select your own exercises in order to work on a specific area of the body, or you can design your own routine.

If any exercise in unclear, consult a physical therapist, sports scientist or your personal trainer to ensure you are doing it correctly. It is always wiser to be overcautious rather than undercautious when it comes to keeping the body fit.

Just remember that no exercise should cause pain — a little discomfort maybe — *but not pain*.

The body tends to know only what is familiar and not necessarily what is right; it loves to avoid the exercises that are a little more difficult. This may be your chance to change this!

1

Understanding the Body

Before we start analyzing muscles and discussing muscle fitness, we need to understand what structures that body comprises. This section will review the major systems of the body. These include the cardiovascular, respiratory, gastrointestinal, lymphatic, nervous, craniosacral and musculoskeletal systems. The focus in the second half of this chapter will be on the musculoskeletal system as this is the most important system to understand in relation to muscle fitness.

The Major Systems of the Body

The basic unit of the body is the cell, which exists in all shapes and sizes. It is within the protoplasm, or jelly-like substance of the cell, that complex biochemical changes occur, creating the processes of life as we know them.

Groups of cells that perform similar functions are referred to as tissue. Examples of tissue are muscles, nerves and the connective tissue that separates and supports these structures. These tissues in turn form organs such as the heart, lungs, glands and skin, and the skeleton. Organs and tissue with similar functions form the body's main systems.

All the structures of the body receive oxygen carried in the blood through arteries from the heart. This enables them to function. The veins then pump the used blood back to the heart. This system of blood flow is called the *cardiovascular system*. Your pulse rate (the rhythmic pumping of the arteries) is an indication of the efficiency of your heart. For normal healthy individuals, the slower the pulse rate the fitter they are.

The *respiratory system* refers to the lungs and airways. We breathe in oxygen and exhale carbon dioxide. (Plants, alternatively, utilise carbon dioxide to stay alive and exhale oxygen.) When resting, we breathe air in at eight to twelve breaths per minute. This air, which is rich in oxygen, is then taken by the heart and pumped throughout the body in the blood.

The *gastrointestinal system* includes all the structures involved in the digestion of food. The stomach, small and large intestines, pancreas and liver are all part of this system. These organs are often referred to as viscera.

The *lymphatic system* is the system responsible for fighting infection and comprises very thin vessels that carry a clearish fluid. Nodules called lymph nodes may be found at certain places, mainly in the armpit and the groin area. Infection causes these to enlarge.

Another system, the *nervous system*, consists of the brain, spinal cord and nerves. The latter carry messages to the muscles, organs and viscera. Nerves emerge from in between each vertebra off the spinal cord, which is a direct extension of the brain.

The *craniosacral system*, a less well known system, refers to the cranium (the skull) and how it is linked up with the sacrum (the base of the spine). Fluid flows up and down the spinal canal and cushions the brain within the skull. This fluid is called the cerebrospinal fluid and is produced in the brain. It is pumped up and down the spine at a regular rate of six to twelve beats, or cycles, per minute. This pulse is not easily detectable by the individual, but it can be palpated anywhere in the body by a skilled craniosacral therapist.

All these systems work together to keep the body functioning as an efficient machine. No one system can go wrong without having an effect elsewhere in the body, either directly or indirectly, in the short or long term. It is almost as if a chain reaction occurs. For this reason the body can be viewed as a closed *kinetic* system; that is, it is continually changing, adapting and altering due to both intrinsic (the body's actual systems) and extrinsic (outer environmental) forces.

The Musculo- skeleton System

Let us consider in more detail the system that is most important to sporting activity, which is the musculoskeletal system. This system comprises the *skeleton* (bones) and the muscles.

The skeleton

Basically, the body is a bundle of bones — 226 altogether. Bones are important because they provide attachment for our muscles and a stable structure for supporting our organs as well as our muscles. The skeleton consists of a group of long bones in the arms and legs, for movement; shorter and smaller bones in the hands and feet, for maneuverability; the vertebrae of the back and the bones of the pelvis, which provide support; and lastly, the rib cage and the skull, which protect the body's vital organs.

Bones are linked together in various ways at the joints. All joints are stabilized by the ligaments, which act like strong elastic bands. The major types of joints are ball and socket (e.g. the shoulder and hip) and hinge (the knee). Other joints are sliding (the wrist and ankle), pivot (the first cervical vertebra at the base of the skull, which rotates around the second cervical vertebra) and the vertebral joints that connect the vertebrae of the spine. The vertebrae are cushioned and separated by cartilaginous discs, providing shock absorption for the spine. Figure 1.1 shows details of the skeleton and the spine. In our limbs most joint surfaces (e.g. knee, elbow, and shoulder) are protected by cartilage and fluid. These are called synovial joints.

All joints have an *active* range of movement made possible by the muscles that contract around the joint, and a *passive* range of movement. *Range of movement* simply refers to how far we can move a joint. An active range of movement is how far we can move a joint consciously by contracting our muscles, such as when we raise our arms above our heads. A passive range of movement is the extra movement that takes place in a joint that we cannot consciously control, but which can be achieved by a therapist. Techniques such as mobilization and manipulation, preformed by trained health professionals, can be used to achieve passive range of movement of joints. Injury to muscles usually results in stiffness due to loss of, or reduced, passive joint range in underlying joints. Until both active and passive ranges of movement are gained, stiffness in a joint may be felt, or an injury may recur.

The muscles

In most parts of the body there are layers of muscles. Larger muscles tend to be towards the surface while the smaller muscles are usually found in the deeper layers, providing stability for joints and for further refining gross (larger) movements. For example, the short deep muscles in the back provide stability between each vertebra when we bend forwards to lift heavy objects, while the larger, more superficial muscles contract through a much greater range. When exercising, it is important to stretch and strengthen all muscles through their full range, as daily activities rarely do this, and adaptive shortening of the deeper muscles can occur. This in turn can cause the stiffness we start to feel as we age. Regular stretching, and strengthening, and improving our posture, can minimize this effect.

Obviously it is impossible to review all the 450 muscles in the body in a book of this size. Figure 1.2, however, shows most of the superficial muscles as well as some of the more important muscles in the deeper layers. When you are learning new stretches or strengthening exercises, try to feel the area being worked and think of which muscle you are using.

Movement Terms and Anatomical Positions

Specific terms are used to describe how muscles move the body. These terms can be applied to movement at any joint once the body moves from the resting anatomical position (a standing position with the hands resting by each side). Following are definitions of the main movement terms:

Flexion A movement that makes the angle between two bones at their joint smaller, for example, when the arm is moved forwards and up in relation to the body from the shoulder joint. For the trunk, the term 'flexion' means bending forwards.

Extension The opposite action to flexion, which occurs when a limb is straightened. For the trunk, 'extension' refers to bending backwards.

Abduction A movement away from the middle of the body, such as when the arm is lifted sideways away from the body.

Adduction A movement towards the middle of the body, such as when the arm is returned closer to the body after being abducted.

Rotation A movement in a circular direction.

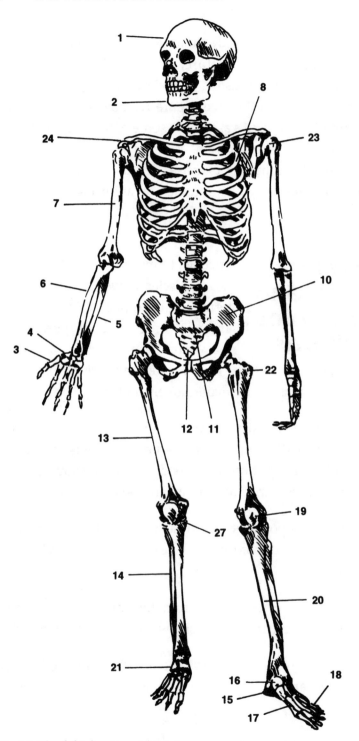

Fig 1.1 *The skeletal system and spine*

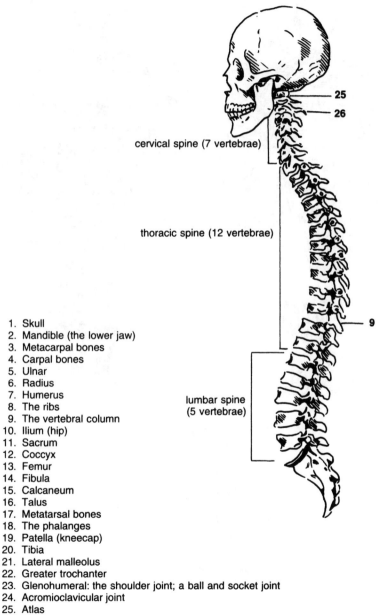

cervical spine (7 vertebrae)

thoracic spine (12 vertebrae)

lumbar spine
(5 vertebrae)

25
26
9

1. Skull
2. Mandible (the lower jaw)
3. Metacarpal bones
4. Carpal bones
5. Ulnar
6. Radius
7. Humerus
8. The ribs
9. The vertebral column
10. Ilium (hip)
11. Sacrum
12. Coccyx
13. Femur
14. Fibula
15. Calcaneum
16. Talus
17. Metatarsal bones
18. The phalanges
19. Patella (kneecap)
20. Tibia
21. Lateral malleolus
22. Greater trochanter
23. Glenohumeral: the shoulder joint; a ball and socket joint
24. Acromioclavicular joint
25. Atlas
26. Axis
27. Tibiofemoral joint; the knee joint; a hinge joint

Major muscles of the front

Major muscles of the back

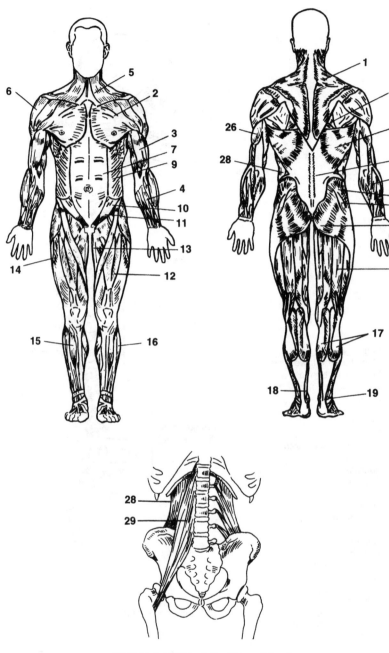

Deeper muscles of the hip and back

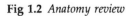

Fig 1.2 *Anatomy review*

1. Trapezius — has 4 parts. The upper fibres shrug the shoulders upwards, while the middle and lower fibres pull the shoulder blades together towards the spine
2. Pectorals — rotate and pull the arm inwards and across the body
3. Biceps — bends the elbow and rotates the hand upwards with the thumb turned out
4. Forearm flexors — bring the palm of the hand onto the forearm
5. Neck flexors — pull the head and chin forwards onto the chest
6. Deltoid — has 3 parts. The middle fibres raise the arm away from the body, the anterior part moves the upper arm forwards and the posterior part moves the arm backwards
7. Rectus abdominis — an abdominal muscle that flexes the trunk and is responsible for lifting the head and shoulders upwards when doing a sit-up
8. Forearm extensors — consist of a number of muscles, which extend or bend the wrist backwards
9. External oblique — abdominal muscle that turns the trunk at an angle and is used when doing oblique sit-ups
10. Internal oblique — an abdominal muscle that lies under the external oblique and works with this muscle when doing oblique sit-ups
11. Transverse abdominis — an abdominal muscle that pulls the abdomen in. The abdomen protrudes when doing a sit-up if this muscle is not working effectively
12. Quadriceps — consists of 4 muscles. The rectus femoris (a) on the front of the thigh flexes the hip and extends (or straightens) the knee, while the others, the vastus lateralis (b), vastus medialis (c) and vastus intermedius (d) extend the knee only
13. Adductors — a group of 4 muscles that move the leg inwards and across the body
14. Iliotibial band — a tendinous extension on the outside of the thigh, which assists with rolling the femur inwards
15. Tibialis anterior — a muscle on the front of the shin that pulls the ankle back towards the body and assists in maintaining the arch of the foot
16. Peroneals — turn the outer part of the foot up and out
17. Gastrocnemius — bends the knee and helps you to stand up on your toes (called ankle plantarflexion) in a toe raise
18. Soleus — assists the gastrocnemius with toe raises
19. Achilles tendon — an extension of the gastrocnemius that inserts into the heel bone
20. Hamstrings — a group of 4 muscles. The biceps femoris (a) has 2 parts, both on the outer side of the femur. They extend the hip, flex the knee and turn the knee outwards. Semitendinosus (b) and semimembranosus (c) lie on the inner side of the femur. They extend the hip, bend the knee and turn the knee inwards
21. Gluteus maximus — the large buttock muscle that extends the hips and turns the thigh outwards
22. Gluteus medius — moves the thigh outwards away from the body. It works hard when we stand on one leg
23. Hip external rotators — a group of 6 muscles that turn the thigh and hip outwards
24. Latissimus dorsi — often called 'swimmer's muscle', this extends the spine backwards, in addition to pulling the arm downwards and inwards after it has been raised above the head
25. Rhomboids — 2 muscles that keep the shoulder blades close to the spine. With poor posture and rounded shoulders they are very weak
26. Triceps — straightens the arms at the elbow after it has been bent
27. Back extensors — this group includes both superficial and deep muscles. Most run from the base of the spine (the sacrum), take attachments from each vertebral level and run through to the neck (cervical spine). Each of these muscles has a slightly different role, but between them, they provide stability for us to stand upright. When contracted, they extend (or arch) the spine backwards and some side-bend or rotate the spine
28. Quadratus lumborum — side bends the trunk
29. Iliopsoas — an important hip flexor that works actively when we are in a sitting position

When describing an exercise the following terms (anatomical positions) may be used:

Superior Towards the head.

Inferior Towards the feet.

Anterior Front, or in front of.

Posterior Back, or at the back of.

Medial Towards the middle of the body.

Lateral Towards, or on the outside of the body.

2

Knowing the Facts
on Muscles

Our cardiovascular fitness is determined by the efficiency of the heart and lungs, but our body shape and tone are influenced directly by our muscles. Therefore, an integral part of obtaining a higher level of overall fitness is understanding the muscles. This chapter discusses various muscle types, muscle structure, what determines the shape of muscles and how they are physiologically able to move the body during exercise.

The Importance of Muscles

Muscles cover ligaments, bones and joints, and permit movement by shortening or contracting to pull our bones into motion. They also provide shape to our skeletal frame. In any sporting activity hundreds of muscles are playing their part. Smooth and cardiac muscles ensure the flow of oxygenated blood around the body to provide nutrients to the working or skeletal muscles, which are able to move the various parts of the body required for any particular sport.

Types of Muscles

A muscle is an elastic structure that supports, protects and permits movement in the body. Muscles may differ in length, shape and size. Within our body they comprise at least 40 per cent of our body weight. Dependent on their function, muscles are divided into three basic types: skeletal, smooth and cardiac.

Skeletal muscles include the arm, leg and back muscles, and are associated with voluntary movement of the body (controlled by us at will). If we wish to move our leg or foot, for example, electrical impulses are sent from the brain via the nerves, and these activate the relevant muscles. There are over 450 skeletal muscles in the body.

Smooth muscles are found in the stomach and arteries and are associated with involuntary movement. These muscles work continuously even when we are asleep. The smooth muscles permit the arteries to pump the blood flow away from the heart, and the veins, also under involuntary control, pump the used blood back. Keeping fit will improve the efficiency of these muscles, and will therefore improve our overall circulation.

Cardiac muscles are those found in and around the heart. These are also associated with involuntary movement and work continuously to keep the heart pumping. The fitter we are, the more efficiently our heart is able to work.

The Structure of Muscle

All muscles are made up of smaller filaments called myofibrils. On a microscopic level some of these filaments are thick and some thin. The former are called myosin and the latter, actin filaments. Figure 2.1 illustrates the relative size of these filaments in relation to the muscle. A bridging, locking mechanism, which prevents the filaments from disengaging once they get to a certain length, permits motion of each muscle within a certain range. When we stretch regularly we can achieve an improvement in the resting length of a muscle. If we don't stretch regularly, the muscles will shorten, resulting in muscle stiffness. Long-term poor posture is the result of shortened (and weakened) muscles.

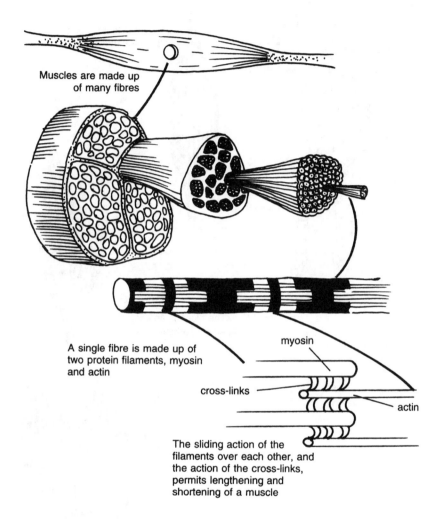

Muscles are made up
of many fibres

A single fibre is made up of
two protein filaments, myosin
and actin

myosin

cross-links

actin

The sliding action of the
filaments over each other, and
the action of the cross-links,
permits lengthening and
shortening of a muscle

Fig 2.1 *Muscle structure*

Muscle Shape

Skeletal muscles are usually one of three different shapes. These are: unipennate, such as the rectus femoris (in the thigh); bipennate, such as the biceps (in the upper arm); and multipennate, for example, the deltoid (at the top of the shoulder). See Figure 2.2.

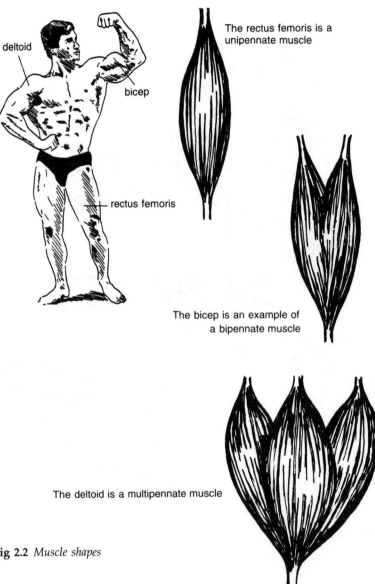

deltoid

bicep

rectus femoris

The rectus femoris is a unipennate muscle

The bicep is an example of a bipennate muscle

The deltoid is a multipennate muscle

Fig 2.2 *Muscle shapes*

Muscle Action

The action a muscle performs is determined by a number of factors. The most important of these are where the muscle starts, called its origin, and where it finishes or attaches to the bone, called its insertion. The length of the muscle, the type of joint it overlies and the direction in which its fibers run (i.e. its shape — see Fig. 2.2) determine the specific action a muscle performs. Muscles may overlie one, two or a number of joints, permitting different actions for the one muscle.

A concentric contraction occurs when two ends of a muscle are brought closer together, and an eccentric contraction occurs when the two ends move apart. An isometric contraction is when the length of a muscle does not alter but is placed against a resistance, for example, the forearm muscles isometrically contract in an arm wrestle.

Muscles may work as individual units or with surrounding muscles to perform a particular movement. The main muscle used to move a joint is called the agonist, or prime mover. Muscles assisting the action are called synergists. While these muscles are working, other muscles may be required to stabilize the joint to permit the movement. These stabilizing muscles are called fixators. Muscles that relax and lengthen to permit a movement are called antagonists. Smooth sporting action may become inhibited if agonist, antagonist imbalance exists. For example, tight back extensors (muscles that run the length of the spine) may inhibit the abdominal or stomach muscles from contracting effectively when doing a sit-up — often called an abdominal crunch.

3

Answers to Questions about Muscles

Exciting advances in sports science in the 1980s have provided new answers to many of the old questions regarding muscles, exercise and fitness. However, depending on whom you are speaking with, you will often get very diverse answers to the same question.

This chapter addresses the more commonly asked questions on muscles, and attempts to sort fallacy from fact. One of the main areas of confusion relates to weight loss and exercise. Many people take up exercise programs in order to lose weight, but are discouraged to find that, even though they look better, the scales register weight gain. This chapter explains how this can happen.

How do muscles work?

Muscles are like ropes; they exert forces by pulling rather than pushing. Similarly, muscles cannot lengthen themselves; they can only relax and contract. When a muscle contracts, it moves a joint and when it is relaxed, the body does not move. Some skeletal muscles, however, are contracting at a very low grade level all the time. Our deep back muscles are an example of this. These muscles tend to tighten and need stretching regularly. So your back muscles, for example, always need more stretching than the abdominals (these usually need strengthening because they are relaxed too often!).

What happens to muscles with age?

Skeletal muscles are either postural or phasic, depending on their function. With age, postural muscles — those that support us in standing, sitting and lying — tend to tighten, while phasic muscles — those that are more active when we are in motion — tend to weaken and lose tone. Examples of postural muscles are the calves, hamstrings, back extensors, iliopsoas (a hip flexor) and pectorals in the upper limb. Examples of phasic muscles are the quadriceps, abdominals and tibialis anterior. However, the way in which we stand will determine how our muscles are used. That is, muscles that should be postural may not be used properly and therefore may not have the tone they should have.

Unfortunately, all muscles do tend to lose tone as we age. The supportive connective tissue and fascia that surrounds, interconnects and supports muscles and other body structures loses its elasticity. After the age of thirty this process usually becomes more noticeable. However, by maintaining good posture we can retain healthy tone in our muscles and hopefully decrease the impact of gravity on our bodies, which causes our muscles to sag. With age, muscles that are not used regularly not only tend to lose tone but also accumulate fat. This often happens in the abdominal and thigh areas. It must be noted though that fat deposition is influenced by other factors, such as diet and hormones. For instance, women, possibly for childbearing reasons, gain fat on the thighs and buttocks, while men, for unknown reasons, tend to gain fat on the stomach.

In summary, it does seem that the key to slowing down the

ageing process is a combination of regular exercise, stretching and sound nutrition.

Is it too late to get fit after the age of fifty-five or sixty?

Almost any person, irrespective of age or physical condition, can benefit from exercise. The older you are though, the more important it is to take precautionary measures; and if you are recommencing a fitness program, you should have a medical check-up. Whatever your age, do take care to respect your body's limits.

Are muscles of women and men the same?

While the basic physiological properties of muscles are the same for both sexes, more general aspects of body composition differ, creating the visible differences between males and females. The three significant body differences to note are strength (and size), fat content and flexibility.

Strength

It would be easy to assume that men are stronger than women, particularly as they generally have larger muscles. Because of the male hormone testosterone, men do tend to bulk — that is, increase the size of their muscles — more readily than women, especially when they engage in a weight-training program. However, a muscle's size does not accurately indicate its strength. Furthermore, when men and women participate in regular exercise, the results are interesting. Research indicates that when women undertake weight training there is minimal difference between the strength of men and women, measured in proportion to body weight. On the other hand, without strength training, women's strength is generally found to be 25–28 per cent lower than men's.

Women often worry that they might bulk if they use weights, but, unless they have a higher than normal level of testosterone, they will increase both their strength and tone with weight training, but will not bulk significantly. The taking of steroids will obviously create undesirable bulking — for both sexes.

Fat content

Women have a generally higher content of fat in their bodies. The average fat content for a young, healthy adult man is 10–15 per cent, while for a young, healthy adult woman it is 16–25 per cent. As men and women age, they have 5–10 per cent more body fat than their younger counterparts. However, the increase in body fat with age is not solely physiological; it is also lifestyle related. Physical activity and level of fitness directly influence body fat content.

Approximate levels of fat content can be measured by fat calipers, used by specialists who do fitness testing. A more accurate figure can be determined by underwater weighing, but this is usually available only at sports science research laboratories.

Flexibility

As a rule, women tend to be more flexible than men. While female hormones are claimed to contribute to this, and bearing in mind that we all have our own skeletal and anatomical limitations, men can improve their flexibility. However, in later years it becomes more difficult to improve flexibility for both sexes. Physiological changes in connective tissue contribute markedly to the stiffness that occurs with age — far more so than sex-related reasons. In other words, the more we exercise and stretch, the more chance we have of reducing the predisposition we have to becoming stiff and tight in our joints and less flexible as we age.

The main difference in flexibility between the sexes is most obvious during pregnancy. Due to the presence of the hormone relaxin in the female body, ligaments become lax, predominantly in the pelvic region, the hips and the lower back. This is why it is important to maintain strength throughout pregnancy — swimming and walking are excellent. Likewise, after birth, ligaments take a few months to regain their normal physiological properties, so postnatal fitness is critical as soon as it is medically recommended. Chapter 9 includes exercises ideal for the new mother.

Are children's and adults' muscles the same?

The basic molecular and physiological structure of adults' and children's muscles is the same. What obviously differs is the ability of children's muscle to grow and lengthen as the underlying growth plates in the bones alter, permitting growth in height. One marked difference between adults' and children's musculoskeletal systems is the relative elasticity of children's tissues. Ligaments, which support joints, do not reach maturity till late adolescence. This means children tend to be more flexible than adults — or at least, should be! Similarly, the connective tissue (the non-contractile part of a muscle) is less fibrous and has more fluid when we are younger. Damage to any of these soft tissues also repairs more quickly. It is not normal for a child to be stiff and inflexible, but being introduced to excessive flexibility work as a child can cause problems in later life.

Are growing pains in children real?

Controversy still surrounds the answer to this question. A suggested reason for growing pains is an imbalance in the rate of growth of the bone compared with the rate of muscle growth. Bones grow more quickly than muscles, which in turn grow more quickly than the sheaths around nerves. This difference in rate of growth between each of these structures is very apparent when children go through a growth spurt; that is, when they are growing at a rate much quicker than normal. Remember though, pain is the body's way of telling us something is wrong, so do not ignore a child's complaints.

Often children may complain of pain in their joints. If it is knee pain, it may be because they are doing too much jumping or running for their age, and the quadriceps tendon (the muscle down the front of the thigh) is pulling on the growth plate of the tibia (shin bone). A large lump may appear just below the kneecap. If this occurs, seek advice and treatment from a sports specialist. It must be attended to as early as possible to prevent musculoskeletal problems in later life.

Children who complain of lower back, hip or feet pain may have a skeletal problem such as leg length difference or flat feet, or a muscle imbalance where a scoliosis (curvature of the spine) or hyperlordosis (often called a sway back) may develop. A postural assessment from a physical therapist and recommended exercises will lessen the predisposition children may have to developing problems later in life.

Referral to a podiatrist (a specialist who deals with feet problems) may be necessary if you notice your children developing strange habits when they are walking, or if they excessively wear down one particular part of their shoes. Corns and bunions on children's (and, of course, adults') feet are a certain sign of imbalance further up the body — usually in the knees, hip or spine.

Whatever the reason, growing pains usually *are* real. If the ache is specific to certain muscle groups, particularly of the weight-bearing joints, muscle tightness, weakness or imbalance may be present. A postural assessment from a health practitioner will screen for this. Weight bearing — that is, standing, sitting, running and so on — actually stimulates the growth of bone. Therefore, it is unusual to have growing pains in the upper limbs. The exception is in teenage girls who may suffer thoracic (mid-upper back) pains as their bust is developing. The poor posture that often results at this age is very difficult to correct later on, so this is the time to subtly assist the teenager to become aware of the principles of good posture.

Consult a doctor if a child complains of generalized aches throughout the body. It may not be a problem of musculoskeletal origin.

A final point with children is that genetics do play a part in determining body type, but only to an extent. Features such as being tall and thin, short and plump, bow-legged and so on are not easy to alter. (See Fig. 3.1.) However, intervention in the teenage years can minimize the tendency for children to adopt their parents' postural habits, such as stooping forward or slumping, as posture tends to be learned rather than inherited in many instances. Therefore, it is probably ineffective to try to alter a child's posture if the parents' stance is not good!

Why do some people seem to have strong muscles, while others cannot seem to build up their muscles, no matter how much they weight train or exercise?

Some people do tend to be more naturally musclebound than others. The scientific term for describing how a muscle appears and feels is 'muscle tone'. Two major factors influencing both muscle size and overall muscle shape are body type and muscle tone. Both of these are clarified below.

Body type

Our body shape may be classified into one of three groups: *ectomorph* (tall and thin), *mesomorph* (muscular), and *endomorph* (a tendency to be short and plump). See Figure 3.1.

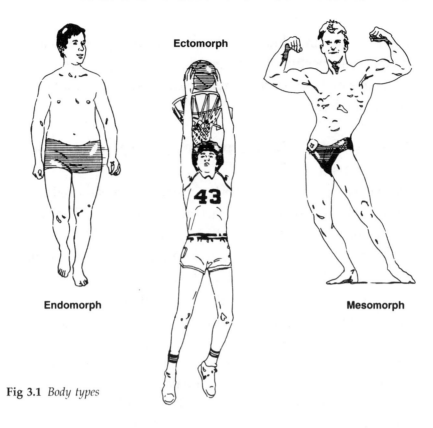

Fig 3.1 *Body types*

Most of us have attributes from each body type, but in general it is more difficult for a tall, thin person to build up muscle bulk just as it is difficult for an endomorph to achieve unnatural slimness. Being realistic about our body type will assist us in determining our long-term goals with respect to exercise and sport. For instance, short, plump people do not make good basketball players. Fortunately, as a rule we tend to choose sports suitable for our body types.

sports suitable for our body types.

Muscle tone

The tone of a muscle (or its 'tautness' or 'firmness') is determined not only by body type but also by how we use our muscles. A tall, thin person who stands poorly may have a protruding stomach, flat, toneless hamstrings and calves, and a poked-forward chin. He or she may look plump, but it is simply poor posture that creates this effect. Corrective postural measures and appropriate exercise can restore good tone to all these muscles.

Will exercising my muscles improve my posture?

Poor posture means that the body not only looks tired, but is also vulnerable to neck and back ache, and injury. The type of work you do, sporting activities, your personality and emotional state, heredity, height, and pain or disease are some of the major influences on your posture.

Being fit doesn't necessarily mean you will have good posture. In fact, many exercise program can lead to tight muscles tightening, weak muscles becoming weaker and strong muscles becoming even stronger. Therefore, the key to achieving ideal posture is maintaining a balance of strength and flexibility between muscle groups. Though each individual is different, Figures 3.2 and 3.3 illustrate the main components of poor and ideal posture with respect to muscle balance.

Participating in a regular aerobic fitness program, doing the exercises shown in the daily routines to achieve muscle balance and a positive outlook will all contribute to a better posture.

Why do I get stiff and sore muscles a few days after exercising?

One fallacy is that sore muscles are due to lactic acid accumulation. Lactic acid is a waste product produced when we exercise but the body removes this lactic acid. Most of it has been absorbed within 20 minutes post-exercise, and within 2 hours, traces of lactic acid are minimal.

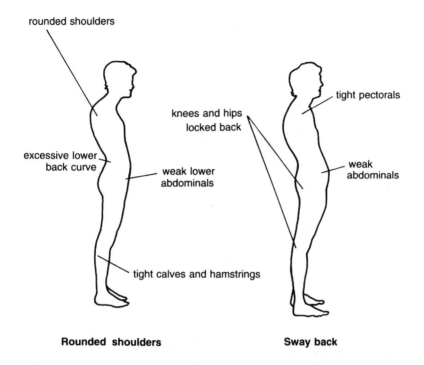

Fig 3.2 *Two types of poor posture, showing areas of weakness and tight muscles*

There are four main reasons proposed for muscle soreness:

1. *The pressure theory* This suggests that post-exercise wastes such as histamines build up in the muscles and cause pressure and therefore pain. Weightlifters tend to support this idea but it has little scientific backing.

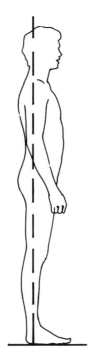

Fig 3.3 *The ideal posture, showing a balance between all muscle groups. An imaginary plumbline should fall through the middle of the ear, middle of the shoulder, middle of the femur and down to slightly anterior to the ankle front*

2. *The spasm theory* This claims that ischemia (pooling of blood), which is caused by exercise, results in the production of a pain substance (substance P), which in turn causes further pain. The evidence supporting this idea remains contradictory.

3. *The tear theory* This proposes that pain is caused by microtears in muscle fibers following unaccustomed movement. However, examination for chemicals in exercised muscles, which could be indicative of tears, has shown that these chemicals exist independently of pain.

4. *The connective tissue theory* This is perhaps the most scientifically supported theory of muscle pain. It is based on the observation that soreness is most common following negative (eccentric) muscle contractions, rather than positive (concentric) muscle contractions. Research indicates that negative contractions put a greater strain on a muscle's non-contractile components (the connective tissue). Microtears in the connective tissue, as opposed to the contractile muscle fibers, are thought to cause the pain.

None of these reasons has been conclusively proven but the most scientifically accepted one is the connective tissue theory. It is important to note here that stretching prior to, and at the completion of, exercise reduces post-exercise soreness. Stretching is particularly beneficial when doing unfamiliar exercise, as this is more likely to result in muscle soreness.

Does regular exercise lead to arthritic joints?

Many people believe that exercise will have ill effects on the joints of the knees and back. The good news is that all the research to date indicates that people who exercise regularly are less likely to develop degenerative conditions such as arthritis because of the improvement in circulation throughout the body generally. Rather than damaging bones and joints, running and other forms of aerobic exercise add strength to the bones and improve the nutrition to the joints.

Why do I weigh more after I take up a fitness program?

This aspect of muscle fitness often causes great concern for those who take up an exercise program to lose weight. The simple explanation for this phenomenon is that muscle weighs more than fat. Therefore, people embarking on an exercise program will probably lose overall body fat content, but if they stand on the scales they will weigh more. Scales are therefore not a very accurate measure of our true weight as they do not take muscle size into account.

If I stop exercising, will muscle turn to fat?

Contrary to popular belief, nothing will change muscle to fat (or fat to muscle). Muscle and fat are two different types of tissues. Aerobic exercise (see p. 32) burns up fat and builds up muscle. If you stop exercising and maintain the same food intake, muscles will weaken and lose tone, and your body will start to store excess (unused) calories as fat.

If we carry fat deposits on specific areas of our body, is it possible to spot reduce?

The answer to this is definitely 'no'. By exercising a specific muscle we can increase its tone and strength, but the only way to lose fat from a specific area is to participate regularly in aerobic exercise and reduce overall body fat content. So if you have a large protruding stomach, sit-ups will not reduce its size, but merely give you a firm, strong stomach! As mentioned previously, hormonal and postural factors do influence where we deposit some of the fat in our body.

Is it possible to lose weight by dieting alone?

Although many people diet to stay slim, it is now well known that dieting alone will not lead to weight loss. Most people who go on a weight-reduction diet invariably give it up, and subsequently regain the lost weight (and often more). If you go on and off diets constantly over a period of time, your body's metabolism will slow down in order to cope with the times you are eating less. Therefore, when you are off you diet, your body will store fat more readily, and in terms of muscle/fat ratio you will in effect be fatter.

Regular exercise is definitely more effective than dieting, if you are seeking to lose weight. Aerobic exercise increases the muscles' ability to absorb oxygen, and with regular exercise the body draws on its stores of fat and uses these for energy. An additional benefit is that with regular exercise the overall body metabolism is increased for up to 24 hours after a workout. In other words, even when you are not exercising, you are burning more calories than you would be if you had not exercised!

Do vibrator belts rub away fat, and will saunas help me to lose weight?

Vibrators may provide a little massage and relax tight muscles, and are certainly harmless, but they do *not* rub away fat.

After a sauna, scales may indicate that you weigh less but this is because of fluid loss. The effect is negated once you increase your fluid intake again.

4

Starting an Exercise Program

Probably the most effective way of keeping the body and its muscles fit is to improve cardiovascular, or heart and lung, endurance. There is no means of exercising the heart, lungs and blood vessels directly, but regular exercise results in more oxygen being taken into the body, which increases the efficiency of the cardiovascular system. Every cell in the body requires oxygen to function. The stronger the heart and the more elastic the lungs, the more efficiently the cardiovascular system delivers oxygen. The efficiency of our heart and lungs has a direct bearing on how fit we feel.

If you are not used to exercising regularly, this chapter provides guidelines that will help you to decide what activity is appropriate for you, and for how long and how often you should do it. If you are over thirty and have not exercised for some years, it would be sensible to see your doctor for a medical check-up before commencing a regular exercise programme. This is particularly important if you lead a sedentary or stressful lifestyle, or if you are overweight. Whatever your age and condition, it is advisable to gain some idea of your current level of fitness.

How Do I Know How Fit I Am?

Physical fitness is defined as having enough energy to perform your daily duties with energy left at the end of the day to enjoy your leisure time. While this is a non-scientific definition, it describes an accurate way of assessing your individual fitness.

On a more scientific level, measuring your heart rate via your pulse can be a helpful way of assessing your cardiovascular fitness. As you gain fitness, your resting heart rate should decrease. The ideal time to take your heart rate is first thing in the morning. Place the third and fourth fingers on the side of the neck, where the carotid artery pulse can be detected easily.

The average heart rate for a sedentary man is around 72 beats per minute (bpm), while for a woman it is around 80 bpm. Over the course of a day, the unconditioned person's heart may register 50,000 more beats than the conditioned person's heart. Therefore, the fitter you are, the slower your pulse rate, and the more efficient your heart. In the trained athlete the resting heart rate may go as low as the mid-40s to mid-30s bpm. Marathon runners frequently report resting heart rates in this range.

Fitness testing

If you wanted to find out even more about your level of fitness, you could have a complete fitness evaluation by a qualified fitness instructor or exercise scientist. These people are often employed by gymnasiums, and sports science or sports medicine clinics. The evaluation may involve a stress, or submaximal, test using a bicycle or treadmill as an ergometer (the machine you are tested on). These tests are usually more suitable for the elite athlete, as they test the exercising muscle's ability to use oxygen and determine how intensively you can push your body. Tests provided by gymnasiums such as the Harvard step test are sufficient for most individuals.

What you need to decide is whether you wish to know your heart/lung or your muscle fitness. It is always advisable to determine both if you are commencing an exercise program. If you just wish to know your muscle fitness, a postural assessment may be sufficient. This will identify any muscle imbalance influencing your posture and assist you in identifying your areas of weakness (muscles that are tight and so on). Physical therapists or sports scientists who are interested in posture can do this assessment. If you would like to monitor how you are progressing with your fitness program over a period of time, the aforementioned gymnasium tests would be ideal.

Aerobic and Anaerobic Exercise

The most effective form of exercise for long-term cardiovascular fitness is aerobic exercise. This means breathing in air and oxygen continuously to supply the working muscle. During this form of exercise, there is adequate time for the exercising muscle to utilise the oxygen taken in with each breath. Examples of aerobic exercise include jogging, walking, swimming and some aerobic dance classes. Anaerobic exercise, on the other hand, does not utilise oxygen, but uses energy stores from within the muscle, for instance, glycogen. Sprinting is an example of anaerobic exercise. Have you noticed how a sprinter breathes heavily at the end of a race? A jogger rarely does this at the end of a run, as oxygen is available throughout the jog because of its lower level of intensity.

While both forms of exercise are excellent for fitness, aerobic exercise is essential for improving physical fitness in the long term. The heart and lungs are stressed continuously over a longer period of time, so their efficiency improves. As mentioned, the efficiency of the heart and lungs determines our general level of fitness. Anaerobic exercise is usually performed in short bursts and contributes more to specific fitness for each sport. To be able to perform well during anaerobic activity, however, you have to improve your basic level of aerobic fitness. For instance, if you play tennis socially and decide to combine this with a regular aerobic walking program, you will not be so tired after your social tennis games. You will be aerobically fitter, and therefore able to cope with the anaerobic exercise much more easily.

FITT Aside from having a check-up there are a few basic hints to follow when you are trying to get fit. Using the letters *FITT* we can outline the main things you need to consider when taking up an exercise program.

Frequency

To gain cardiovascular fitness, you need to exercise a minimum of three to four times each week. It is best to exercise every second day as opposed to exercising for a few days and then doing no exercise for the rest of the week.

Intensity

You need to exercise at 60–80 per cent of your maximum heart rate (MHR) to achieve a cardiovascular training effect. Your MHR can be estimated by subtracting your age from 220. The fitter you are, the higher the percentage of your MHR it is safe to work at.

For instance, if you are forty years old and very unfit, you need to work at approximately 60 per cent of your MHR. This would be between 106 and 110 bpm (0.60×180). If you are working at greater than 80–85 per cent of your MHR, you are more likely to be working anaerobically. This is because there is not enough time for the oxygen breathed in to pass from the lungs to the exercising muscle, and the muscle must therefore utilize energy stores from within the muscle. It is difficult to sustain this level of exercise for extended periods of time. To achieve a general level of cardiovascular fitness, aerobic exercise performed at 60–80 per cent of your MHR is advised. To supplement your training, anaerobic exercises are recommended. It is the lower level, sustained exercise that achieves weight loss, if this is your goal, not the high-intensity, high-speed workouts performed in short bursts. The latter form of workout is important to include, though, if your particular sport or activity requires anaerobic work. If you are uncertain as to what level you are exercising at, take your carotid artery pulse for 10 seconds. (Trying to maintain contact for the entire 60 seconds is often difficult if you are exercising.) Once you have a figure, multiply it by 6. This will give you an idea of what range of the 60–85 per cent of your MHR you are working in. The 'whistle' test is another helpful way of assessing whether you are working out at too intense a level. This involves whistling or talking while you jog or walk. If you cannot, you are probably working at too high a heart rate and may be working anaerobically.

Type

As stated previously, to gain long-term cardiovascular fitness, you need to choose an exercise that works you aerobically, such as jogging, brisk walking, cycling and swimming, and some fitness, dance, step, circuit-training or aquarobics classes. The key to working effectively aerobically is to maintain a continuous workout; that is, if you are doing lap swimming, you must minimize the breaks you have between laps and aim for consistency in your workout.

The main influence on your choice of exercise is whether you enjoy it. You may like to vary your exercise routine by combining swimming, jogging and tennis, for example. Alternatively, you may prefer the routine involved in doing just one particular activity. Your choice of exercise will also be influenced by what you can fit into your daily lifestyle. Be realistic

— starting a swimming program in the middle of winter is not a good way of staying motivated.

Time

To be effective in your workout you need to maintain your elevated heart rate for a minimum of 15–20 minutes. In anaerobic activities it is physically impossible to sustain a high level of workout continuously for this length of time. Ideally, you should work out for about half an hour so that you can include a warm-up and cool-down in your exercise routine.

5

Preparing and Training for Sport

Now that you understand the importance of cardiovascular fitness for maintaining general muscle fitness, and know which type of exercise is the most effective, this chapter provides tips that will help you to prepare for and gain full enjoyment from your sport or exercise activity.

Whether you are going for a brisk walk, swimming or having a social hit of tennis, the body needs to be warmed up for the activity. In cold weather, would you turn on your car and drive off without letting it warm up? Your body is similar to a car in this respect. Prior to any sporting activity it needs to be prepared, and at the completion it also needs attention. An adequate warm-up can decrease the risk of injury and improve your sporting efficiency, while a cool-down can reduce the risk of chronic injuries developing.

Warm-up

This should include a loosening of all the major muscles and limbs in the body, whether they are being used in your particular sport or not. Large circular and swinging movements of the arms and a brisk walk or light jog is a helpful general warm-up. Stretching is also essential for loosening stiff muscles and joints prior to sport.

The time spent on your warm-up should correspond to the length of time you wish to spend exercising. If you are going for a 15–20 minute slow jog, a 5 minute warm-up, stretching the muscles you are about to use (quadriceps, hamstrings, calves, hip flexors and lower back), would be sufficient. While you are warm at the end of your jog, a longer stretching session that includes both the muscles you used and those you did not would be ideal. For sports or activities of longer duration, a more extensive warm-up would be recommended. For instance, for an 80 minute Rugby match, 15–20 minutes should be the minimum time spent stretching and warming up.

Cool-down

After sport it is equally important to take a few precautionary measures — particularly to avoid post-exercise muscle soreness. Most sporting activities use some muscle groups more than others. All muscles, both used and unused, must be stretched out at the completion of exercise. This will also reduce your risk of injury next time you exercise.

The intensity of your activity will determine the length of your cool-down. For instance, after a 45 minute aerobics class, a 10 minute cool-down and stretch is adequate. However, when you are warm after exercise, you will find it much easier to stretch, so it is a good idea to spend a little longer with stretches for all body parts if possible.

Training Tips

The three aspects of fitness

Whatever your sport, it is important to consider all aspects of physical fitness in your preparation and training. Usually these are called the three Ss. These are:

Stamina

This refers to the cardiovascular component of your sport. Are the demands of your sport aerobic or anaerobic, or does the sport combine both? Lack of stamina, particularly in contact sports, can lead to fatigue and an increased risk of injury.

Strength

Does your sport overdevelop the dominant side of your body? If so, you need exercises to balance this effect. Do you have adequate strength for your activity? Maybe an increase in strength would improve your sporting performance. With any strength training, try to use weights in a similar range to how you use the muscles in your sport.

Suppleness

Regular flexibility exercises are essential to maintain the suppleness in our joints, ligaments and muscles and will enhance sporting performance. Chapter 6 discusses this aspect in more detail.

Specific skills

Not only should you attend to each of the above, but in training you should also practice the specific skills required by your sport. Following are a few specific training tips:

Change of direction activities

You need to practice agility skills, change of direction activities and stop/start maneuvers, if this is required in your sport. For example, for all codes of football, shuttle sprints, gradually increasing the pace and distance, are an ideal form of specific skill training. For volleyball or skiing, the body must be prepared for change of direction activities, otherwise it is vulnerable to injury.

Duration and nature of specific skills

You need to practice both physically and mentally (i.e. mentally rehearse) the specific skills required in your sport. When practicing first serves for tennis prior to a match, for example, aim for accuracy at a slower speed first, then progress to a few harder serves. If your sport requires a lot of jumping activities, these skills must be practiced in your training and included in your warm-up.

Intensity

Try to train at an appropriate intensity for you sport. Do not just do 3 mile slow jogs if you wish to compete in a 15 mile fun run that you know will be run at a faster pace. Incorporate some 10 and 12 mile runs into your pre-fun run training.

Range of movement

Ensure you achieve the full active and passive ranges of movement for your sport so that the other parts of your body are not overloaded. For example, if you are round-shouldered, you may be tight in the front shoulder muscles and limited in shoulder range. If this is the case and you are a tennis player, when you serve, other parts of your body (e.g. your lower back) will try to compensate. Flexibility training specific to your sport is critical in order to avoid injury.

Balance, rhythm and timing

Have you practiced skills at match pace in training? For example, for basketball, have you practiced long-shot, 3 point goals as well as difficult shots under the basket at close range?

Progression

Are you progressing in your training program gradually? A too rapid increase in training pace, distance or intensity can cause injury.

Staying Motivated

Many people take up a fitness program with zest and enthusiasm but within a few months have abandoned it. The usual reason given is that they have lost interest, suffered an injury, are too tired to keep it up or simply do not have the time to do the activity regularly. One of the problems when people take up a fitness program is that they set unrealistic goals and choose activities they feel they *should* do, rather than those they feel are fun and enjoyable.

In his book *The Sport Drug* (Allen & Unwin, Sydney, 1982), Gary Egger proposes three phases you may experience when you take up any fitness program.

1. *The Discomfort Phase* This is the initial stage when you know you should exercise but your body and mind are telling you differently.

2. *The Physical Phase* This is where you find you can physically exercise more easily — for example, when you are jogging you can go further with greater ease — but your mind still considers the activity a chore.

3. *The Addicted Stage* This is when you cannot go a day without exercise. It is possible to be either positively or negatively addicted to exercise. A positive addiction is when you exercise regularly and feel better for it in all areas of your life. Exercise becomes a negative addiction when obsessiveness sets in. At this stage, one day of no exercise will result in the individual experiencing withdrawal symptoms, such as depression, lethargy or loss of appetite — to mention but a

few! Obviously, the ideal is to find a balance so that exercise is having a beneficial effect on your lifestyle.

How Much Exercise Is Enough?

It is possible to exercise too much. With the upsurge of interest in sport during the 1980s, there has been a corresponding increase in injuries. Many injuries could have been prevented if the necessary precautions had been taken, while others occurred because people did too much exercise, and their bodies were unable to cope. Injuries falling into this category are called overuse injuries.

How much exercise is enough and how much is too much? This is not an easy question to answer, as every individual and his or her respective needs are different. The answer lies in common sense. If you are waking up each morning feeling tired and exhausted, and having to walk down the stairs backwards because you are too sore to walk straight down, it is highly likely you are overexercising!

Unfortunately, for some individuals, their exercising is their income, so rest is not possible when they are tired or sustain an injury. Fitness instructors are classic examples of this syndrome. Employees and employers should give consideration to this when terms of agreement for employment are being negotiated. Fatigue is a prime precursor to injury for the fitness instructor, so look after even the most minor injuries to prevent a chronic problem developing.

6
Stretching

Stretching is an important part of muscle fitness. If we don't stretch our muscles regularly, they may tighten and shorten. (Fortunately, only some of our 450 muscles tighten; otherwise, stretching would take a long time!) Tightened muscles can lead to muscle imbalance in the body, which invariably results in poor posture. This in turn can place stress on various parts of the body, in particular the neck and back, and it may also affect the efficiency of other body systems. For instance, weak shoulders and shortened chest muscles can cause rounded shoulders, a sunken chest and an excessive curve of the mid-back. As well as resulting in neck or back pain, these postural faults can make it very difficult for the individual to breathe effectively.

The Benefits of Stretching

At different times during the day, most of us tend to do some form of spontaneous stretching, because our bodies don't like to be kept in one position for a long period of time. However, this infrequent spontaneous stretching will not improve your flexibility; it simply feels good. On the other hand, taking a break from a fixed position *and* doing specific stretches, repeated regularly, will improve your flexibility, as well as relaxing your muscles and making you feel less tired at the end of the day.

Improved flexibility means that joints can be moved through a greater range. This can enhance sporting performance. Regular stretching combined with keeping fit aerobically may also prevent or alleviate the pain associated with tightened muscles. When you injure yourself — for instance, if you strain a hamstring — the sooner you are able to commence stretching (always working within the limits of pain), the sooner you will recover and return to sport.

In addition, stretching improves blood supply to the muscles and coordination between muscle groups, and decreases the muscle-tightening effect that occurs with age. What's more, it is fun to do.

If you practice the stretches shown in this book, your improvement in muscle tone and general flexibility should soon become self-evident.

The Difference between Stretching and Strengthening

Stretching refers to the elongation that occurs when the origin and insertion of a muscle are moved as far away as possible from each other. Stretching improves the flexibility of the muscle and permits more mobility in the underlying joint. In contrast, strengthening refers to when the muscle is repeatedly contracted against resistance, either through range or within a fixed range. This may cause enlargement of the muscle belly, called hypertrophy. Strengthening may be achieved by working the body against gravity; for instance, by raising the head and shoulders off the floor to strengthen the abdominals when doing a bent-leg sit-up, or by using specific weights.

In all fitness programs there should be a balance between stretching and strengthening. As the role of strengthening in a fitness program is well understood, this chapter focuses on the importance of stretching, which is often neglected.

The Stretch Reflex

When a muscle is suddenly stretched, a reflex comes into play that causes the muscle to involuntarily contract. This is known as the stretch reflex. If you were to suddenly stretch again while the muscle was contracted, you would damage the myofibrils of the muscle, causing microtears, which result in fibrous or scar tissue. This is the main reason that bouncing while stretching (e.g. bouncing while touching your toes) is not advisable. Not only is it considered harmful to the muscles of the lower back, but it may also stress the discs of the lumbar region of the spine.

How to Stretch

There are basically five types of stretching:

1. *Static stretching* This takes the muscle to the end of its range and, when the position is held for the minimum 6–10 seconds, actually inhibits the stretch reflex. Therefore, the muscle relaxes and permits more range and an increase in muscle length. Static stretches should be repeated about three times, each time moving gently into a new range. Breathing out as you are stretching the muscles assists the body to relax and improves the effectiveness of the stretch. The longer a stretch is held, the more effective the increase in muscle length.

2. *Dynamic stretching* This refers to faster movements where the muscle is gradually worked to its full range. Dynamic stretching is often used in dance, gymnastics and the martial arts. It would also be appropriate for a full-back in Rugby Union. It would be ineffective for this player to simply do static stretching of the hamstrings prior to play. To prepare the leg muscles for the high kicks required in this position

of play, the player must gradually take the hamstrings to their full range. This is done by dynamically stretching them at an increasing speed, but *not bouncing* the movement at the end of range. A dynamic stretch of the hamstrings could be achieved by bringing the bent knee up to the chest initially, while standing, then progressing gradually to straight-leg high kicks.

3. *Ballistic stretching* This refers to fast, jerky movements, where a double bounce is performed at the end of range of a movement, such as bouncing when touching your toes. This type of stretching is not recommended for most sports because of the potential tearing of myofibrils it may cause. In the long term, the tearing only serves to reduce the effectiveness of the stretching because of the scar tissue created. Dancers and gymnasts may incorporate some ballistic stretching into their routines, as their sports require these fast, full-range movements. However, ballistic stretching should be performed in a controlled manner, just short of the end-range of a movement. For all other sports, it is not recommended.

4. *Proprioceptive neuromuscular facilitation (PNF) stretching* This type of stretching has been shown to be the most effective way to increase muscle length. It involves doing a static stretch, followed by an isometric contraction (see p. 15) of the muscle against a resistance — your own hands or a partner's — for 6–10 seconds. Then the muscle is relaxed and gently taken into its new range. It is best to repeat this about three times. Sometimes this stretching is called contract/relax, or hold/relax, stretching. The following precautions should be observed with PNF stretching:

   • It should only be attempted after a total body warm-up.
   • The isometric contraction should never be explosive (i.e. started suddenly).

- A partner should only provide resistance in the isometric phase, and guide rather than force the muscle in the static stretch phase. The person stretching, not the assistant, should take the muscle into its new range.
- The isometric contraction should involve a gradual increase in effort in the first 2 seconds, which is then sustained for an additional 4–6 seconds.

5. *Range of movement stretching* This type of stretching simply refers to taking a muscle through the full range that the underlying joint permits. It is part of the overall concept of Tai Chi and Feldenkrais exercise movements (see Glossary). Working with a practitioner skilled in these forms of health disciplines is an ideal way to learn these movement patterns.

PNF and range of movement stretching are considered to be the most effective forms of stretching. Fast, jerky ballistic stretching is not recommended as it can cause damage to the muscle because of the stretch reflex. Try the different methods to find which form of stretching works best for you. Work with a partner whenever possible, and relax and enjoy your stretching.

Over-stretching

It is possible to stretch too much. Over-stretching can cause laxity in the ligaments that protect the joints. If you regularly experience muscle soreness after a stretching session, you are probably overdoing it. However, if you do enjoy doing a lot of stretching (greater than 1 hour per day), then you must balance this by doing strengthening exercises through full range. This should prevent ligament laxity developing. For most sports, unless you compete at an elite level, static and dynamic stretching should take up no longer than 10–15 minutes of both your warm-up and cool-down (though you can alter this time in accordance with the time spent playing sport).

Hypermobility, or overflexibility

Have you noticed how some people are able to touch their toes, even put their hands or elbows on the floor, while you are struggling to touch your knees? While it may seem wonderful to be so flexible, it does have its disadvantages.

When someone is more flexible than normal, he or she is called *hypermobile*. (Some people call this person double-jointed, but it is anatomically impossible to be double-jointed.) With hypermobility, because of increased muscle length and ligament laxity, the joints can move much further than normal. Some people are hypermobile in all their joints, while others have specific joint hypermobility. The latter usually occurs at the wrist (the fingers can be bent back onto the forearm), or the thumb (it too can be brought back up onto the forearm). It may also occur at the elbows and knees. Both are able to extend past 180 degrees, which is considered to be the normal range at these hinge joints. (This is called hyperextension.)

Specific joint hypermobility normally poses no problems, although occasionally it can if it occurs at the knees. If, when you stand, your knees tend to curve backwards and lock back, try to bend them slightly. Otherwise, postural problems in the spine can develop as the upper back attempts to compensate for this excessive mobility in the lower limb.

General hypermobility should not be a problem, and can be of benefit to a gymnast or dancer. However, if you do not exercise regularly, but have inherent general hypermobility, instability around joints can develop. When young, this may not be a problem, but with age, if strength in the muscles is not retained or if excess weight is carried, stress on joints can be far greater than it is for the inflexible person. An analogy would be trying to drive a car after loosening all the bolts that keep the tires secure. Just as this would be risky, so is our body vulnerable when excessive joint mobility, usually due to ligament laxity, is not balanced by adequate strength.

The reasons for hypermobility are not fully understood. The type of sport or physical activities we are exposed to as children appear to influence our flexibility as adults. For instance, if you did gymnastics or ballet in your adolescent years, your chances of being flexible (but not necessarily hypermobile) when older are greater than if you did no stretching or flexibility work.

However, if you return to sport after neglecting it for some years, hypermobility may be a difficulty, as you will not have the same strength you had when younger. Clunking joints, particularly hips, may be indicative of muscle imbalance or instability in a joint, and this often occurs in hypermobile people. The good news is that hypermobility need not be a problem, but certainly, if you are hypermobile, retaining strength of all muscles is critical to maintaining stability around your joints.

7

Exercises for Each Part of the Body

This chapter outlines stretching and strengthening exercises for all the major muscles and muscle groups of the body, starting with the neck and shoulders, working down to the trunk (which includes the abdomen and back) and then finally the lower limbs, which include the hips, thighs, calves and feet.

Guide to the Exercises

When you perform the stretches, you should feel the muscle or muscles being stretched. If you cannot feel the stretch, you may not be doing the exercise correctly or it may be an inappropriate exercise for you.

Strengthening is important to provide stability around all joints. You should be aware of and feel the muscle you are strengthening. You should not perform the exercise so quickly that you are using momentum to achieve the movement. Perform the exercise slowly and with control.

Both stretching and strengthening are important to achieve balance around our joints. No individual muscle should be stretched excessively or laxity about a joint on one side will result. Do not avoid the exercises that are difficult to do as these are usually the ones you need most!

If an exercise is working a particular muscle, this is stated, but many of the exercises are a combination of movements, involving a few muscles. The shading on some stretches indicates where you should feel the exercise. The arrows indicate the direction in which you should move your body.

Stretches

Hold all stretches for 6–10 seconds at a minimum. Relax and breathe out as you move into the stretch. Do not ease back too far before repeating the stretch. Repeat a minimum of three times. For tighter muscles, try to hold the stretch for longer.

Push to the point of discomfort but do not push through pain. *No exercise should produce pain.*

Strengthening exercises

Start with four to six repetitions (less will be noted in parentheses if this is necessary). Progress to eight to ten repetitions. When this becomes too easy, do three sets, or use an elastic band or weight to increase the effectiveness of the exercise. Remember that quality movement will achieve far more than exercise performed with poor form, in large quantities or at high speed.

Mobility exercises

Some exercises combine stretching and strengthening throughout the range. Start with two to three repetitions of these exercises and progress to four to six. All mobility exercises should be taken to as full a range as your body permits. You should feel where they are working.

Neck and Shoulders

1 **Neck flexion** — to stretch the muscles at the back of the neck (the neck extensors) (× 2–3). Tuck the chin in and bend the head forward. Relax the shoulders. Interlock the fingers, place the hands on the back of the head and gently press the head forward to increase the effectiveness of the stretch. Tilt the head slightly to the right then the left to differ the stretch.

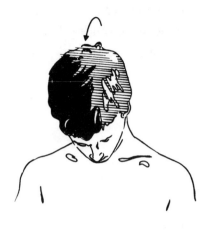

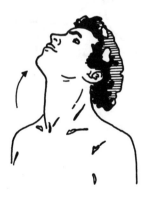

2 **Neck extension** — to stretch the muscles at the front of the neck (the neck flexors) (× 2–3). Look to the ceiling and stretch the neck backwards. Elongate the neck and actively use the muscles to do this; do not just collapse the head back.

3 **Neck rotation** (× 2–3). Look over one shoulder and depress the opposite shoulder. Repeat each side. Do not let the opposite shoulder come forward. Tuck the chin in.

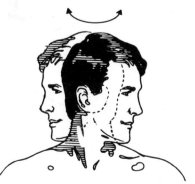

4 **Neck side flexion**
(× 2–3). Pull the ear down to
the shoulder and depress the
opposite shoulder. Do not let
the opposite shoulder rise up.

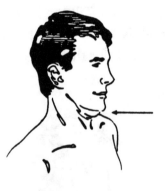

5 **Neck stretch** — excellent
for correcting poor neck posture (× 2–3). Pull the chin
inwards. Create a double chin
and gently look to the right,
then the left. You should feel
the stretch at the side of the
neck. Pull the shoulders down
gently to increase the effectiveness of the stretch.

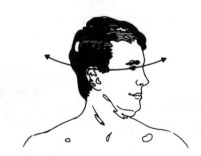

6 **Sitting neck stretch**
(× 2–3). While you are sitting, place your right hand under your buttocks, with the palm faced upwards. Now create a double chin without bending the head forward, and look down to the right knee. Gently bend your trunk towards the left and depress the right shoulder to increase the effectiveness of this stretch. Repeat for the left side of the neck.

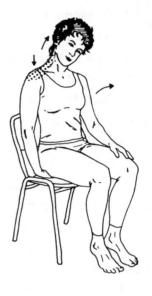

7 **Sitting neck and shoulder stretch** (× 2–3). Sit with your legs crossed, and place your hands on and around the opposite knee; push down with your knees and this will depress your shoulders. Now gently make a double chin and drop your head slightly forward. Now look to the left knee and pull the left shoulder down. Repeat this to the right. Change and cross your hands the opposite way to feel the stretch in a slightly different place.

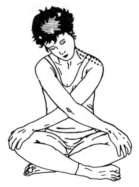

8 **Wall exercise** — excellent for correcting poor posture (X 6-8) First, stand against a wall with your heels 3 to 6 inches away from the wall. Try to flatten your lower back on the wall; a small gap here is fine. Your shoulder blades and the back of your head should be resting comfortably against the wall. If you cannot do this, make this your goal. Now roll the shoulders inwards so that the palms are facing outwards, take a breath in and, as you exhale, raise your arms above the head. Maintain braced and tightened abdominals (stomach muscles) and slightly flatten the back. Your goal is to have the elbows on the wall while maintaining the back close to the wall. Keeping the mid-back against the wall, bend your elbows and slide your arms downwards, to shoulder level, then stretch up again. Now repeat this exercise with hands turned outwards. Repeat each day and you will note an improvement in your posture within a very short time.

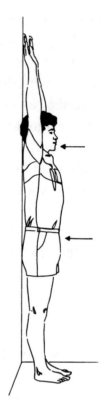

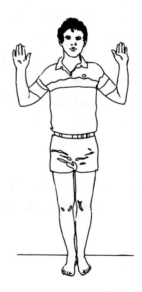

9 **Neck and upper back strengthening** ($\times$ 6–8). Lying face down, rest the arms either side so that the elbows are at the same height as the shoulders and bent at right angles. Lift the head but keep the back of the neck lengthened. Now raise one arm by pulling the shoulder blade towards the spine and downwards. Now lift the other arm. Hold both up for 5–6 seconds, then place both down. Rest. Repeat very slowly.

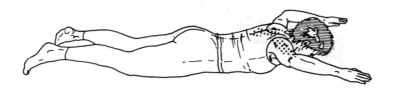

10 **Advanced neck and upper back strengthening** — excellent for correcting round shoulders associated with poor posture ($\times$ 6–8). Commence as in exercise 9 but extend the arms fully outwards beyond the head. Raise one arm slowly, then the other. Relax then repeat. To progress, slowly bend the elbow and bring the hand back to the ear, alternating arms, while maintaining the head off the floor and keeping the back of the neck lengthened. If you are a dancer, this same exercise can be performed with both the neck and back arched into an extended position, maintaining the pelvis on the floor.

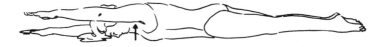

Chest

11 **Pectoral stretch** — excellent for correcting poor posture. On all fours, place the hands with extended wrists out in front, pull the shoulder blades together and let the mid-back drop inwards. Keep the hips directly over the knees and the knees apart.

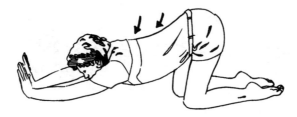

Keep the fingers and wrists extended for a more effective stretch. You may need to commence this exercise by sliding and extending one hand from cat-stretch position (exercises 41 and 42), then doing the other hand, before progressing to doing both hands together.

12 **Chest and shoulder stretch.** On all fours, with the arms extended in front of the body, keep the hips over the knees, and the knees apart. Now place the right hand over the little finger side of the left hand while the wrist is extended, and lean into the outside of the left shoulder. Repeat with the other hand.

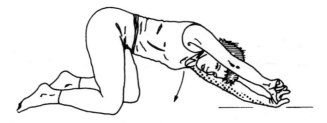

13 **Pectoral and tricep strengthening** — modified push-up, variation I. Using a modified push-up position, with elbows kept close to the sides of the body and hands directly under the shoulders, lower and raise the torso, keeping the head and trunk in a straight line.

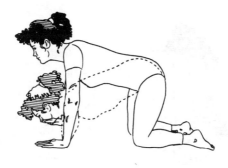

14 **Shoulder girdle strengthening** — modified push-up, variation II. Using the modified push-up position again, as for exercise 13, place the hands wider than shoulder width. Progress to placing the hands further forward to make the push-up harder, but do not let the back collapse inwards as you are doing the push-up. Keep the abdominals tightened.

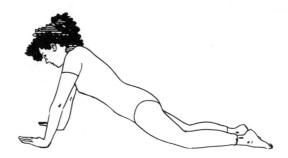

15 **Full push-up** — for shoulder and upper back strengthening. Progress to a full push-up if you are able, and place the hands on top of each other to increase the difficulty of the work on the shoulder muscles. Repeat, using the hand positions suggested in exercises 13 and 14.

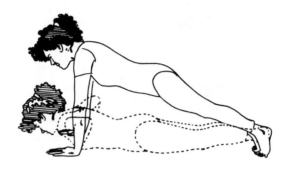

16 **Isometric pectoral strengthening.** Push palms together. You should feel the strain in the chest muscles. Repeat with arms outstretched above the head.

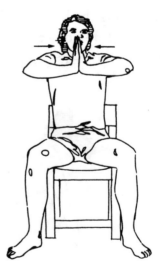

17 **Sitting pectoral and shoulder strengthening** (× 4–5). While sitting on a chair, place hands on either side of the chair, grip, and lift the body weight. Hold for 6–10 seconds.

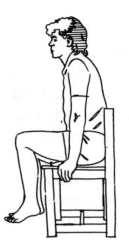

Shoulders, Arms, Upper Back and Mid-back

18 **Mid-back spine and shoulder mobility: using a rod or towel.** Take a rod and clasp it with the palms turned down. Take a breath in as you raise the rod up, and then breathe out as you slowly ease the rod over and behind the body. Keep a wide grip initially, but your goal is to achieve the exercise with the hands placed at shoulder width. Do not arch the back and keep the knees slightly flexed. Do not do this exercise if you have shoulders that dislocate easily.

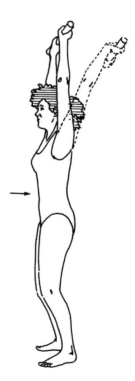

19 **Mid-back and shoulder mobility exercise** — excellent for reducing stiffness in the shoulders and mid-back (× 4–5). Cross the arms and clasp hands in front of the body at shoulder height. Take a breath in and, as you exhale, stretch the hands above the head. As you again breathe in, bend the elbows and bring the hands down behind the neck. Release the hands so that just the index fingers are clasping when the hands are behind the neck. Stretch the arms up again, then repeat, bringing the elbows down again, fingers behind the neck.

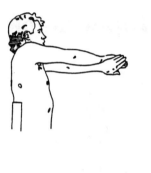

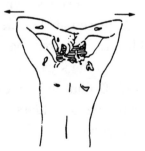

20 **Shoulder mobility** — excellent for the front aspect of the shoulder. Lying face downwards, arch backwards from the lower back, keeping the pelvis on the ground. Rotate the shoulder downwards to the floor by letting the elbow come directly over the hand. Think of pulling the shoulder blade away from the spine. Keep the head facing the floor. Do not rotate the lower back or mid-back. This exercise is not recommended if you have shoulders that dislocate easily.

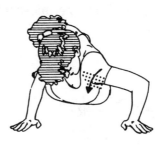

21 **Shoulder and mid-back stretch (thread the needle).** Once on all fours, with knees apart and positioned directly under the hips, thread the right hand under and through so that it is directly beyond the left hand. Now pull back into the right shoulder blade by pushing the back of the hand into the floor and curving the tummy upwards and in. Change the position of the hand to alter the stretch. Repeat on the opposite side. This stretch can be made more effective by making a fist with the hand you are pulling back. By doing this, you should feel the stretch in the back of the shoulder more.

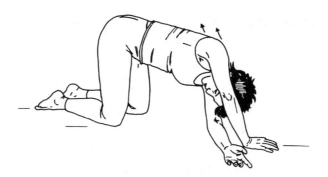

22 **Shoulder and mid-back mobility** — can improve poor posture by increasing mid-back spine extension. On all fours, with the chin resting on the hand and with the elbow bent, weave one arm through and stretch as far down as possible. Now rotate from the mid-back and pull the arm back up and behind.

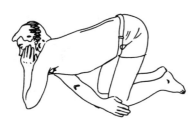

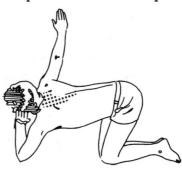

23 **Advanced mid-back stretch.** Commence this exercise from a standing position with legs placed wide apart. Now turn the right foot outwards and keep the left foot facing ahead. Maintaining the trunk in the same plane as the legs, clasp the inside of the right ankle with the right hand. Counterbalance the elbow against the knee and then open the chest by extending the arm upwards. Stretch the fingers as far as they can go, then slowly stretch the arm over the head. This is an advanced exercise; repeat it slowly and with control on the opposite side.

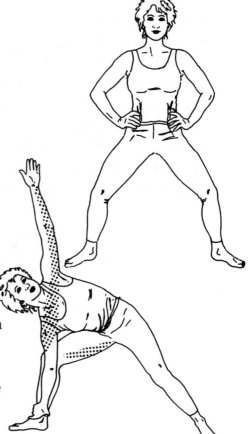

24 **Outside shoulder stretch.**
Place one hand up and behind
the neck. Bring the other hand
up and onto the outside of the
elbow. Gently pull it down.
Increase the stretch by side-
bending to the side opposite to
the arm you are stretching.

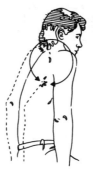

25 **Shoulder rotations: sitting or standing** — for shoulder mobility. Rotate each
shoulder forwards, up and
back. Do not move the chest
upwards. Keep the spine
straight. Now rotate the shoulders in the opposite direction.

26 **Shoulder shrugs** — to
release shoulder tension. Lift
both shoulders up to the ears.
Tighten the shoulder and neck
muscles, then release; now let
them relax again. Do not poke
the chin forward as you do
this. This is an ideal exercise if
you are a student or have a
sedentary occupation.

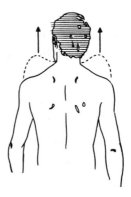

27 **Anterior shoulder stretch.** Start this stretch by placing the hand against a wall, with the elbow close to the body. Rotate the body away from the arm being stretched. Then progress to placing the elbow and forearm up against a door ledge (or an open doorway), keeping the elbow higher than the shoulder. Now take a step forward and rotate away and backwards from the arm you are stretching. Repeat both sides.

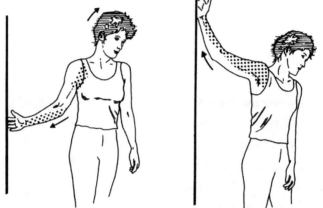

Exercises 28–31 are excellent if you have a sedentary occupation or if your sport involves the wrist or elbows (e.g. tennis or golf).

28 **Fingers, wrist, shoulder and neck stretch (progression from 27).** While standing, place the wrist in an extended position against a wall. Commence with the elbow bent. Then slowly step away from the wall until the elbow is straight. This is a helpful exercise if you get pain in your forearm referring from your neck. Do not do it if your pain is aggravated.

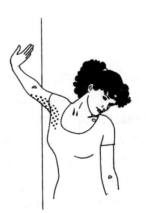

29 **Wrist and finger stretch.**
With arms outstretched, pull
the fingers backwards towards
the forearm. Repeat by stretching the fingers in the opposite
direction onto the back of the
wrist. This is more effective if
you have your arm by your
side, flex the wrist and pull
the fingers up onto the palm.
Vary the angle of your hand
and you will achieve a slightly
different stretch.

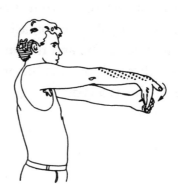

30 **Forearm flexor stretch.** Once kneeling, sit the buttocks
on the lower legs. With the palms of the hands on the mat
and the fingers directed towards the body, try to lean backwards, maintaining the wrists on the floor. Progress by bending the elbows gently. This exercise can also be done with
hands on a table while standing.

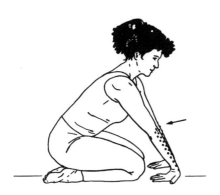

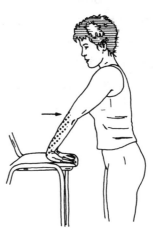

31 **Hands on hips.** Try to rest your hands on your hips, with your palms in contact with your body, and the fingers directed towards the armpits. This is a challenging exercise!

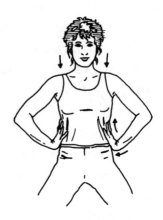

32 **Posterior shoulder stretch.** Bend one arm at right angles, and hold at horizontal level. Place the back of the other hand at the back of the elbow. Counter-resist at this point, then pull the arm across the body further. You should feel the stretch between the shoulder blades. Vary the height of your arms if you cannot feel any stretch.

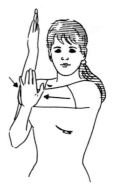

33 **Posterior shoulder and mid-back stretch.** Place the left hand in front, the arm bent at right angles, and hold at shoulder height. Now thread the right arm under and through and try to place the palms together. Push the elbows together and you will feel the stretch between the shoulder blades. Repeat this with the arms around the opposite way, and move the elbows to the left and to the right to vary the stretch.

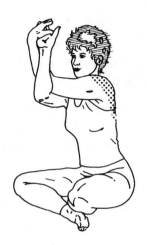

34 **Posterior shoulder and upper back stretch.** Sit with the knees bent and apart, heels together and feet pointed outwards. Cross the arms so that each hand is clasped around the opposite foot. With chin on chest, pull back between the shoulder blades, bend the trunk slightly to the left then the right, while pushing outwards with the feet. Repeat with the arms crossed the opposite way. To increase the difficulty of this exercise, slowly slide the heels away from the body while maintaining the pull on the mid-back and upper back.

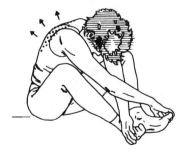

Caution — do not do this exercise if you have a sore lower back.

35 **Upper back stretch.** Sit with the soles of the feet together. Place the hands under the ankles (try to have the elbows as close to the ground as possible) and put the palms on the floor. Push down with the ankles while you pull up between the shoulder blades. Try to think of the top of the head touching 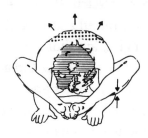 the floor as you are relaxing forward. Slowly move the hands forward, away from the body, and bring the heels closer to the body to increase the effectiveness of the stretch. If you cannot tuck your hands under the ankles and have your elbows on the floor, replace this with exercise 34.

Shoulders and Back

36 **Side trunk and shoulder stretch.** Sitting, one leg bent, with the foot just resting against the inside of the opposite thigh, place the opposite hand on this leg, then bring the other hand over and reach towards the outstretched leg. If you can, clasp the outside of the ankle, look under the elbow and pull up to stretch the side of the trunk. If you cannot reach the outstretched leg, replace this with exercise 37.

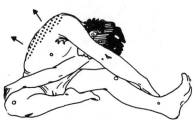

37 **Side trunk and hip stretch.** This stretch can be done by standing adjacent to a wall. Keep the feet parallel to the wall and let the body lean outwards, away from the wall. Tighten, and use the abdominals (not the arms) to move back towards the mid-line.

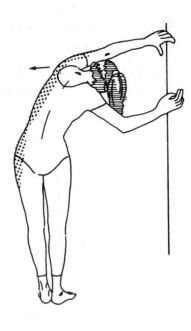

38 **Side trunk, shoulder and hip stretch.** Standing adjacent to a door frame, commence as in 37. Take the arm farthest from the wall and hold onto the wall, cross the same leg behind the other leg, and you will feel a stretch from the shoulder, right through to the hip and outer thigh.

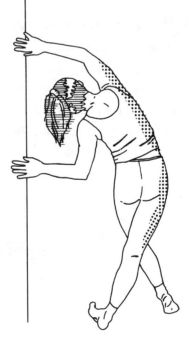

39 **Advanced mid-back spine mobility.** Place both hands on a table at hip height. Aim to pull the shoulder blades together and curve the mid-back inwards. You can bend the knees if the hamstrings are tight.

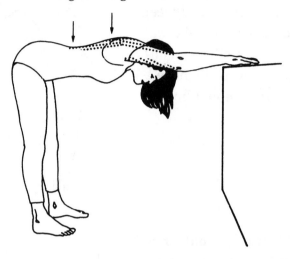

40 **Advanced shoulder and mid-back stretch.** This is a progression from exercise 39. It can be done in a standing or kneeling position. Place the elbows on the edge of a chair and place the palms together. Slowly drop the spine downwards towards the floor. An excellent exercise for releasing the shoulders at the end of a busy day.

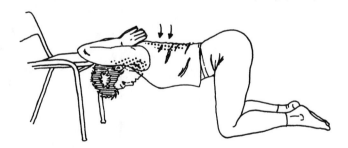

The Back

41 **Cat stretch: extension** — mobility exercise for the spine. Breathe in as you let the spine curve inwards, and pull the shoulder blades together. Keep the knees directly under the hips. Breathe out as you curve upwards. Move gently up then down. Do not hold each position.

Caution — if you have a back complaint, do not let the back drop down past the horizontal.

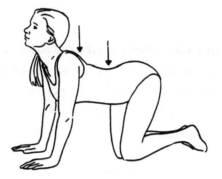

42 **Cat stretch: flexion** — mobility exercise for the spine. See exercise 41.

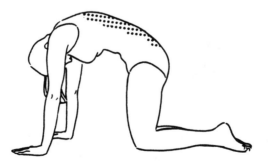

43 **Lower back release** — (× 1 — hold 20–30 seconds). From position shown in exercise 42, keep the hands fixed out in front and stretch from the arms, through the spine, as you slowly place the buttocks between the feet. Be sure to have the tops of the feet touching the floor.

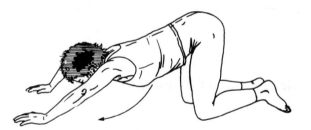

44 **Spinal flexion/extension stretch.** After cat stretch and lower back release, keep the chin close to the floor, while following through into an arched back position. You may need to move the hands forward a little before commencing the second part of this stretch.

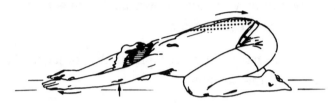

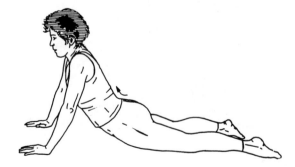

45 **Passive back arch and abdominal stretch** (× 4–5). Keeping the hands under the shoulders and trying to keep the pelvis on the floor, pull the shoulder blades together and let the back muscles relax as you arch back. For the beginner, it is advisable to rest up on the elbows, then progress to straightening the elbows, and gently and slowly arching the back. If you pull your body weight forward and upwards while you are resting on your elbows, you will achieve an abdominal stretch.

Caution — do not do this exercise if your back aches when you lie face down on your abdomen.

To advance this exercise: place the toes on the floor, with ankles flexed, and move the hands closer together under the shoulders. Slowly press up through the shoulders and mid-back to a count of 5, and control your body weight through your arms as you return to resting position (again to a count of 5). This is an excellent exercise for strengthening the shoulders and stretching the back.

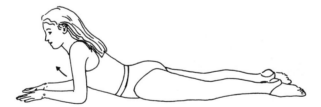

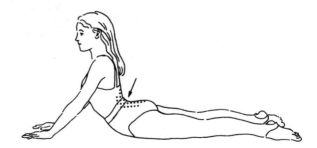

46 **Gentle back release** (× 6–8). Lying on the back with knees bent, feet on the floor, press the small of the lower back into the floor. Hold for 6–10 seconds, then relax. This is a gentle exercise for easing lower back discomfort. Placing a pillow or book under your head will release the neck and lower back even more effectively.

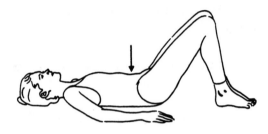

47 **Spinal release stretch.** Hands resting on the knees, lift the feet off the floor. Have the hips at right angles and rotate the knees to the right then the left, slowly and gently. Keep the knees slightly apart and in line with the hips.

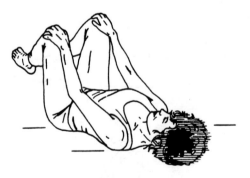

48 **Pelvis and lower back release.** With the hands resting on top of the knees and the feet off the floor, let one leg drop slowly outwards, just short of the floor. Let the other one come over to meet it. Lift the top leg up and over to the other side and repeat. Be gentle and let the exercise flow.

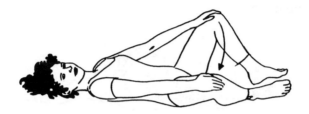

49 **Knee hug stretch** — for the hips, buttocks and lower back. Hug one knee up onto the chest. Progress to bringing the forehead to the knee. Advance by keeping the out-stretched leg off the ground as you stretch each leg. This will strengthen the abdominals as you stretch the hip extensors.

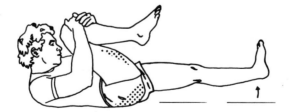

50 **Spinal rotation stretch: lying.** Raise one leg up and over the other one. Place the opposite hand on top of the knee. Gently press it to the floor as you keep the other shoulder on the floor, arm outstretched. Look in the direction of the outstretched hand. Progress to straightening the leg. Increase the effectiveness of the stretch by counter-resisting the knee against the hand.

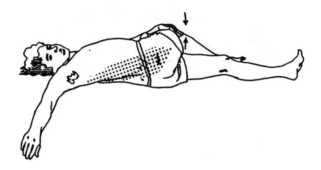

51 **Spinal rotation and hip stretch.** Lying with one leg bent, start by crossing one leg over the other, then let the weight of the top leg stretch the lower leg to the ground. Keep the head turned the opposite way and maintain the arm outstretched.

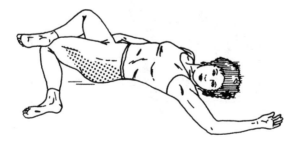

52 **Double leg spinal rotation.** Spinal rotation can also be done with both knees bent up with a rolled towel held between the knees. Rotate both legs one way and then the other. Keep the pelvis on the ground and the feet off the ground.

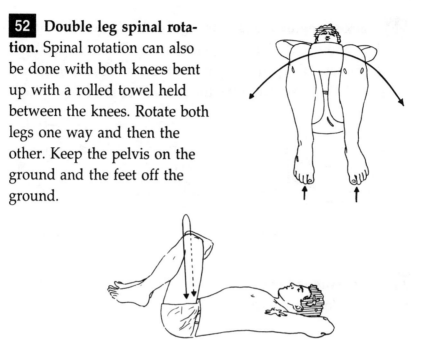

53 **Spinal rotation stretch: sitting.** Place one foot on the outside of the other knee, while this leg is outstretched. Rotate the shoulders past the knee. Gently press the outside of the elbow against the bent knee. Resist and repeat. Rotate a little further, keeping the spine upright. Try to place the hand between the knee and ankle to increase the difficulty of this stretch.

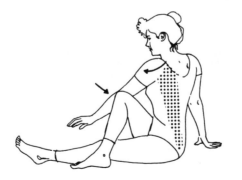

54 **Back-strengthening single leg lift.** Push the pelvis into the floor and use the buttock to lift the leg. Try not to arch the lower back. Only lift the leg 6 to 8 inches off the floor. Keep the ankle flexed and the toe pointed to the floor.

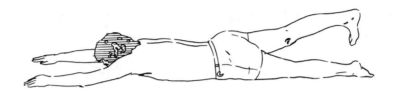

55 **Back–strengthening single arm lift.** Lift the arm. Keep the elbow close to the ear.

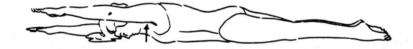

56 **Opposite leg and arm lift strengthening.** Lift the opposite leg and arm but stretch them out long, rather than arching too far. Maintain a double chin and keep the back of the neck lengthened.

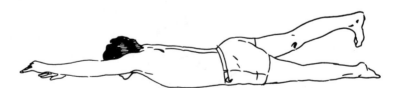

57 **Alternate swimming** — for back strengthening. Try not to arch while bending the opposite foot and arm back towards the head. Repeat each side.

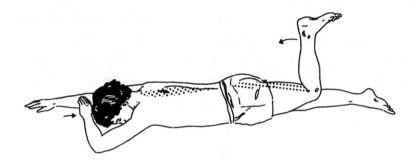

58 **Side trunk strengthening.** Lying on your side with both legs at right angles to the body, lift the head and shoulders off the floor at the same time as you lift the top leg. Try to get the hands to the top of the leg. Keep the knee and ankle parallel to the floor.

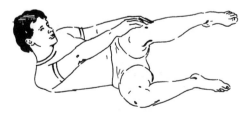

59 **Lower back stretch.** Outstretch one leg and keep the other bent. Keep hands or elbows on the floor if you can, and gently keep moving forward. Hold each position for 6–10 seconds before you stretch forwards. To increase the effectiveness of the stretch, start with the toes pointed, then bring the ankle back into a flexed position. Try to move forward from the lumbar spine, not simply the thoracic (mid-back) spine, which is often already too flexible. This exercise is not recommended if you have rounded shoulders and a forward curved upper back.

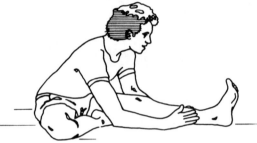

60 **Advanced spinal stretch** (× 2–3). Sit with legs extended, ankles flexed and heels resting against a wall. Place the hands behind the head on the opposite shoulder. Slowly curve the chest in and continue to flex the spine forward. This is a very advanced exercise. Only repeat it once until you know your body is ready to do it.

Caution — Never do this exercise if you have back pain.

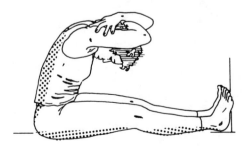

61 **Advanced lower back side trunk stretch.** Sitting with legs astride, ankles flexed, take a breath in and side-bend the trunk while stretching each arm to the opposite leg. Progress to keeping the back straight and leaning forward with the legs still in this position, arms outstretched in front.

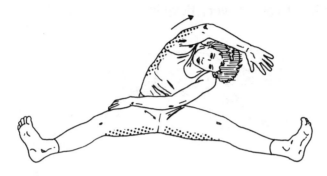

Hips

62 **Hip stretch.** While on hands and knees, push into one buttock, feel the muscles in the buttock give, then stretch a little further into the hip.

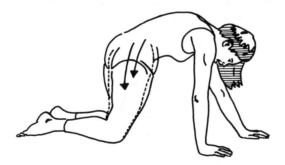

63 **Advanced hip stretch.** From cat-stretch position (exercises 41 and 42), place one leg at 45 degrees to the body, over and behind the other leg. Place the top of this foot on the floor. Let the body weight gently stretch into the hip of the bent leg. Do not just collapse to the floor. This stretch will be ineffective if you are very flexible.

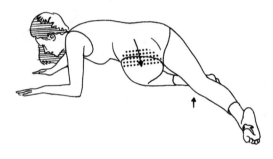

64 **Posterior hip stretch.** This is a wonderful hip stretch if you are wanting a challenge. Place the bottom leg with knee bent so that the heel is not close to the buttocks. Position the top leg (you will need to lift this leg) across so that the heel is resting in the knee crease. Have the ankles at 90 degrees (i.e. flexed). Very gently lean forward, curving the spine inwards (extending it). Move to the left and the right so that you feel all the outer muscles of the hips. Repeat with the legs crossed the opposite way. Start this exercise with legs simply crossed, then progress to the above.

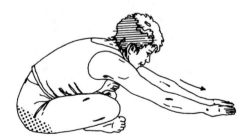

65 **Hip and side trunk
stretch.** Sitting either cross-
legged or in the position
shown in exercise 64, place
one elbow on the ground and
stretch to this side. Repeat
both sides.

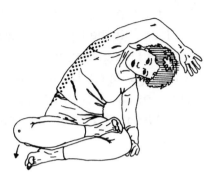

66 **Outer hip stretch.** Place
the leg to be stretched behind
with toes 3 to 4 inches away
from the opposite heel.
Place the outside of the foot
on the ground and let the
body weight fall into this hip.
Do not bend at the hips, but
lean away from the hip you
are stretching, keeping the
upper part of the body in line
with the hips. To achieve a
more effective stretch, take the
leg further across and away
from the other foot. Always
combine this stretch with exercise 68.

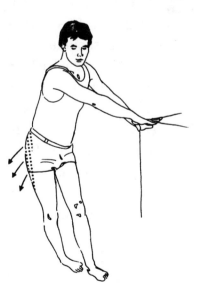

67 **Hip strengthening.** Lie on your side, legs outstretched. Raise the top leg, keeping the toes flexed and turned towards the floor. Lift the leg 25–30 degrees, then turn the kneecap so that it is facing straight ahead and lower the leg. Try not to let the legs touch. Do not arch the back, and keep the shoulders, hips and feet in one line. Use an exercise band around the ankles if you want to increase the difficulty of this exercise.

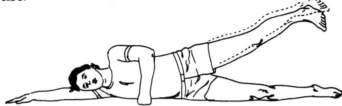

68 **Outer hip strengthening.** Exercise 67 may be done with the top leg bent. This time keep the bottom leg flexed, while the bent knee, shoulder and hip are maintained in a straight line. Do not arch the back or drop the hip or knee backwards. Tighten the buttocks and raise the top leg, keeping the knee slightly higher than the foot. You may need to put a pillow between your knees if this is too difficult initially, and raise the top leg just a little off the pillow. Be careful not to bend at the hip. Relax the leg then repeat by raising the leg 10–15 centimetres above hip height. Lower the leg, then repeat. Keep the knee pointed upwards throughout the exercise.

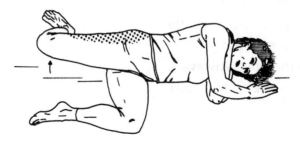

Buttocks

69 **Buttock strengthening** (× 6–8). Lying face down, bend one leg at right angles, push the pelvis into the floor, tighten the buttock and lift the bent leg. Keep the toe flexed and do not arch the back. This exercise can also be performed when on all fours (in the hands and knees position). Rest on the elbows and do not hyperextend the lower back if trying the exercise this way.

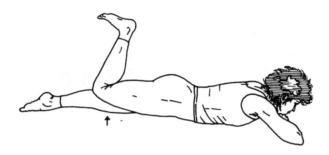

70 **Buttock and upper hamstring advanced** (× 6–8). With one leg bent and the other outstretched, lift the buttocks up, keeping the pelvis horizontal to the floor. If the extended leg is lifted higher, the exercise will be simpler. Repeat slowly with each leg.

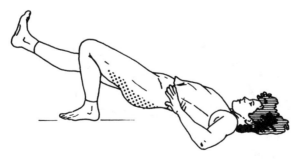

Abdominals

71 **Sit-ups: beginners** — for upper abdominals strengthening. Not recommended if you have rounded shoulders. With knees bent up, tuck the chin onto the chest, and raise the head and shoulders not more than 30 degrees. Tighten the buttocks while you are raising the head and shoulders. Be careful not to poke the chin out and try to keep the head in line with the body as you lift up. Create a double chin before lifting the head and shoulders.

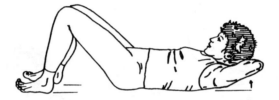

72 **Sit-ups: intermediate.** Doing sit-ups this way will prevent you from hurting your neck and is the most effective way to use your abdominals. Bend the knees, lift the feet, press the heels into the floor, tighten the buttocks and place the hands behind the head on opposite shoulders. With the head cradled in the arms, use the abdominals to raise the trunk. Keep the body in a straight line. You will only be able to raise up 10–15 degrees.

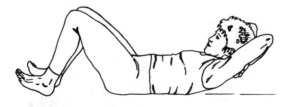

Progression (a) This exercise may also be done with legs extended and outstretched. To protect the back, rest the heel of one foot on the toes of the other. Repeat with the legs crossed both ways.

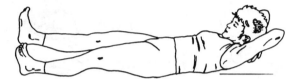

Progression (b) This exercise may also be done with the legs held in the air, and hips at 90 degrees. Oblique abdominals can also be done this way.

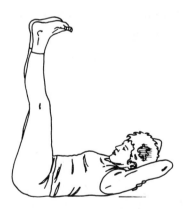

73 **Sit-ups: advanced.** With knees bent, feet flat on the floor, head resting in the crossed arms (as in exercise 72), lift the buttocks off the floor and raise the head and shoulders minimally. This is a very challenging exercise. Do not repeat if it hurts the lower back.

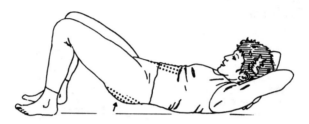

74 **Oblique strengthening.** Starting with knees bent, raise one knee upwards but not towards the chest. Keep the hands beside the head, not under it, with elbows bent. Try to bring the elbow to the knee, not the knee to the elbow. Progress to holding both knees and hips at 90 degrees, keeping the lower back flat, and lift the opposite elbow to the knee. By out-stretching and extending the other leg, you will increase the difficulty of this exercise. Beginners should commence obliques with the feet on the floor.

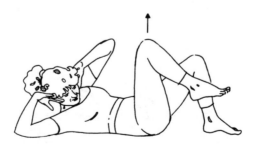

75 **Beginners' lower abdominals strengthening.** Lying on the back, hug one knee onto the chest. Now brace the abdominals (do not just fill the abdomen with air by holding your breath) and raise the opposite leg off the floor, keeping the knee bent. You may need to simulate a cough to locate the lower abdominals. Keep one hand on the abdomen to ensure this muscle works throughout the exercise. Keeping the lower back on the floor, straighten this leg, then bend up again. Initially, you may need to slide the heel on the floor until you can do the exercise with the leg in the air. If this exercise is too easy, progress to exercise 76.

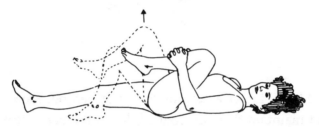

76 **Intermediate lower abdominals strengthening.** Lying on the back, place the hands on the lower abdominals, just inside the hip bone. Tighten and brace. Now lift one knee straight upwards (not towards the chest). Now lift the other leg. Try to hold both up for 4–6 seconds, then relax. If it is too easy, you are probably bringing the knee towards the chest, not lifting it 2 to 3 inches towards the ceiling.

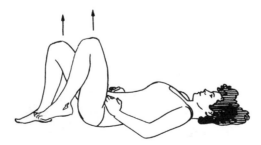

77 **Advanced lower abdominals strengthening.** Once you can achieve exercise 76, progress by extending one leg slowly, ankle flexed, and slowly repeating eight to ten times on each leg. Keep the back flat on the floor. This exercise is also an excellent pelvic-stabilizing exercise.

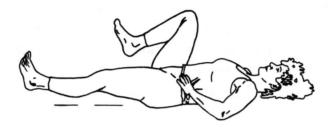

78 **Athletes' lower abdominals strengthening.** Raise both legs and maintain them at right angles to the body. Bend the knees and hip initially as you raise the legs, to protect the back. If you cannot keep the knees straight, do not do this exercise. Push the heels together and flex the ankles. Make eight to ten small circles clockwise (only 4 to 5 inches in each direction), then repeat counterclockwise. This is a very challenging exercise.

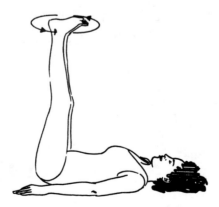

79 **Advanced oblique strengthening.** Progress to letting the legs drop slowly 8 to 10 inches to each side. Use the opposite abdominals (tighten them) to bring the legs slowly back to the mid-line. Now progress to lifting the legs slowly back to the mid-line, then lifting the legs vertically to the ceiling. Keep the ankles flexed and the heels pushed together.

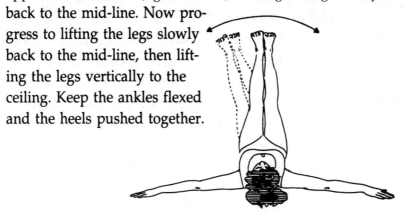

80 **Inner thigh stretch and oblique strengthening.** Lying on the back, both knees bent up, feet on the floor, place the hands on the inside of the hip bone, then let the knee drop outwards to the floor. Use the obliques on the opposite side to bring the knee back to the mid-line by tightening and bracing the abdomen. Do not let the abdomen protrude outwards. Your bracing should have the effect of pulling the abdomen in and flattening the stomach. An excellent pelvic-stabilizing exercise. Progress to doing the exercise with a straight leg.

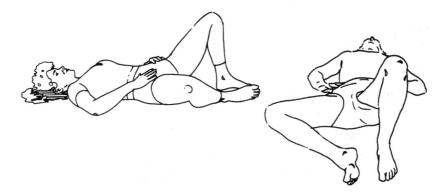

Thighs

81 **Inner thigh stretch: standing/squatting.** Stand with feet astride, parallel to each other. Now transfer your weight onto one leg and drop down onto this knee; feel the stretch on the inside of the thigh. Repeat by turning the foot of the out-stretched leg towards the ceiling. Drop the buttocks closer to the floor if you can. Do not do this exercise in the full-squat position if it hurts your knees. Keep the elbow on the inside of the bent knee and turn this hip out further to increase the effectiveness of the stretch. Counter-resist at the elbow and knee.

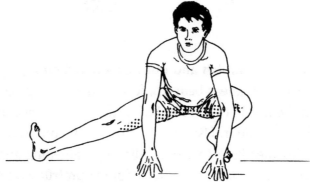

82 **Inner thigh stretch: sitting.** Sit with the soles of the feet together, with the elbows resting on the inside of the knees. Gently counter-resist on the knees, then relax and let the legs stretch closer to the floor. Progress to leaning forward, keeping the back straight.

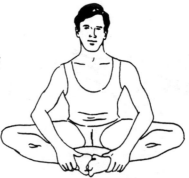

83 **Inner thigh strengthening.** Lying on one side, with the top leg bent up and over the other, raise the bottom leg and repeat. Keep the foot of the outstretched leg parallel to the floor. Start with the head and shoulders on the floor. Progress to lifting the head up slightly, letting it rest on the hand.

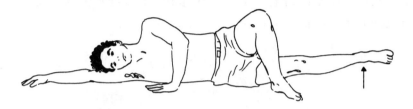

84 **Quadriceps stretch.** Clasp the foot first with one hand, then with the other, and pull the foot towards the buttocks. Keep the knees close together. Do not arch the back or flex the hip. Keep the abdomen tucked in. This exercise can also be done by resting the foot on a chair or fence; usually the other leg not being stretched needs to be bent for this to be effective.

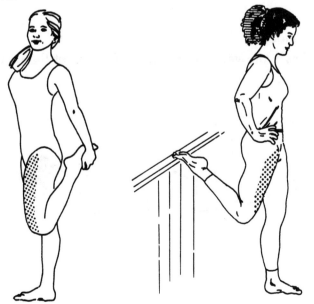

85 **Advanced quadriceps stretch.** Lie on the edge of a (preferably quite high) table, and place one leg over the edge, with the foot flat and knee bent. Now clasp the other foot (or use a towel around the foot) and bring the heel towards the buttocks. To maximize the effectiveness of this stretch, drop the head gently over the end of the table. Be careful to keep the lower back flat on the table, not arched.

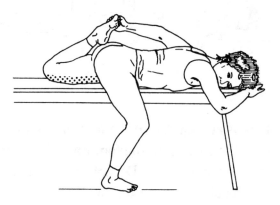

86 **Hip mobility.** Lying face downwards, bend one leg, let it drop slowly outwards and then in. Do not let the pelvis roll.

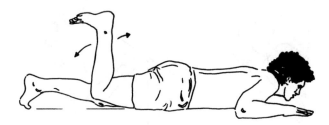

87 **Hip flexor stretch:**
kneeling — for quadriceps and
iliopsoas. This can be done
with or without a wall. Kneeling with one foot behind, and
the top of the foot against the
wall, flatten the back, tuck the
buttocks under and pull the
abdomen up and inwards.
Bend the trunk away from the
side being stretched. You
should feel this in the front of
the thigh and groin. This is an
excellent exercise if you get
anterior hip or groin pain.

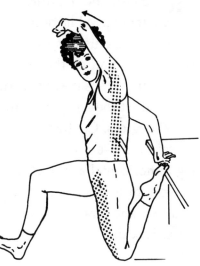

88 **Quadriceps strengthening.** While lying, pull the toes
back. Tighten the thigh and lift the leg. Repeat but do not let
the leg touch the ground when it is lowered. An exercise
band or weight on the foot will make this exercise more effective. Keep the knee locked tightly as you do this exercise. If
an exercise band is being used, bend the knee of the opposite
leg and place the band under this foot.

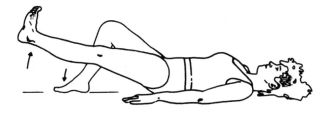

89 **Inner-range quadriceps strengthening.** While sitting with one leg outstretched, place your hand on the inside of the quadriceps (vastus medialis) and let the leg drop down 25–30 degrees. Contract this muscle and use it to raise the leg to horizontal again. Have the foot turned out slightly as you lock and straighten the knee. Flex the foot.

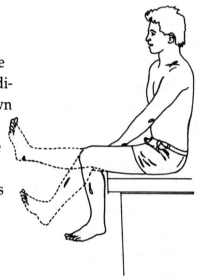

90 **Step strengthening exercise.** Stand on a step and tighten the quadriceps as you bend and straighten the knee. Particularly try to tighten the inside muscle (vastus medialis), as usually this is the weakest of the quadriceps. Use the other leg as a lever by extending it down over the step. Strengthening of this muscle, combined with stretching the hip abductors (exercise 66) and strengthening the outer hip muscle (exercise 68) can assist if you suffer from 'runner's knee' (pain under the kneecap).

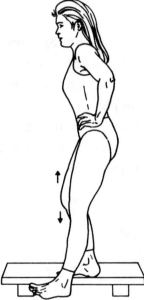

Hamstrings

91 **Hamstring stretch: sitting.** While sitting, curve the lower back inwards and straighten one leg. Try to pull the toes back to stretch tight calf muscles. This is an excellent exercise to stretch the hamstrings if you have a very flat lower back (i.e. you don't have a normal lumbar curve).

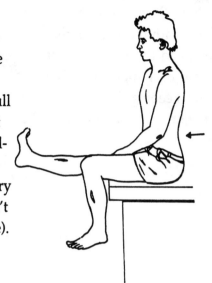

92 **Hamstring stretch: standing.** Lean forward, keeping the back straight. Place one foot in front, pull the ankle and toes back and start with the knee slightly bent. As you lean forward further, straighten the knee and you will feel the stretch in your hamstrings and calf muscle.

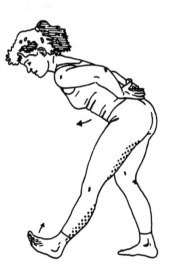

93 **Hamstring stretch: using a chair.** Place one foot on a chair, with the knee slightly bent, and the ankle and toe pulled back (not pointed). Now, keeping the back very straight, lean forward from the hips.

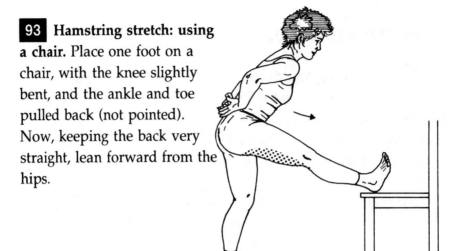

94 **Hamstring stretch: using a fence or table.** Same exercise as 93, but place the foot higher. If you can, place the hand and fingers over the foot and pull the toes back.

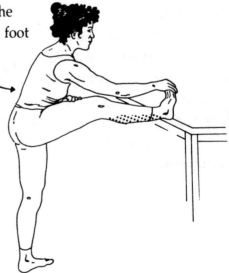

95 **Hamstring stretch: kneeling.** From a kneeling position, place one leg in front for stability. Lean forward, keeping the back straight and the toes and ankles flexed.

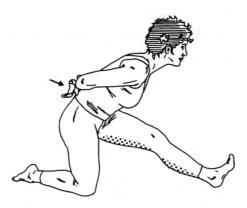

96 **Hamstring and lower back.** With one foot on the inside of the thigh of the outstretched leg, place the hands on either side. Gently try to bend the elbows and ease forward. Do not just curve the head and shoulders forward.

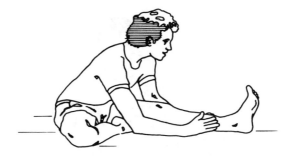

97 **Hamstring stretch: lying.** Bend one knee onto the chest and rest the hand on the back of the thigh. Now try to straighten this leg by placing one hand around the foot and pulling the ankle back towards you. By pulling on the outside and then the inside of the foot, you can alter where you are stretching the hamstring. You may use a towel around the foot to assist with this stretch.

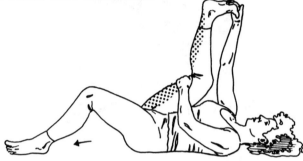

98 **Combined hamstring and inner thigh stretch.** From a full-squat position, come up on the toes of one leg, bend the knee and bring the buttocks towards the floor on this side. Pull the toes back on the outstretched leg and keep the elbow inside the bent leg to provide counter-resistance. Leaning forward with the back straight will increase the effectiveness of the stretch.

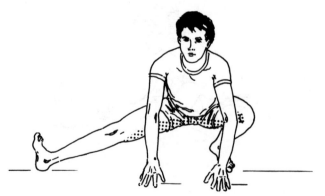

99 **Advanced hamstring and calf stretch.** While kneeling, place one foot up on a stool or chair. Place one hand on the toes and pull them back. Keeping the ankle at 90 degrees, with the knee slightly bent and the back straight, try to lean forward. Put the hand on the inside and then the outside of the foot to alter the stretch slightly.

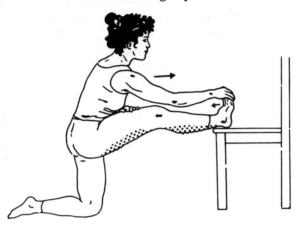

100 **Inner and outer hamstring stretch.** Standing, let the knees bend as you touch your toes. Cross the legs and straighten one leg, then the other. Do not bounce. Repeat by crossing the legs the opposite way.

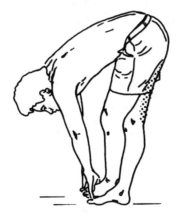

101 **Outer hip stretch.** Place your foot up on a high table with the knee dropped out. Keeping the back straight and leaning forward, you will feel the stretch on the outer hip. This stretch will assist with improving your hamstring flexibility.

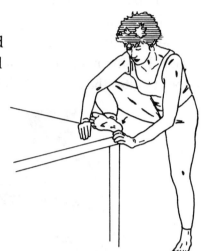

102 **Upper hamstring stretch: lying.** Cross one ankle in front of a bent knee. Now put both hands through and around the bent leg and hug this knee up onto the chest. Counter-resist the ankle against the knee to increase the effectiveness of the stretch. You should feel it at the top of the hamstring and the base of the buttocks.

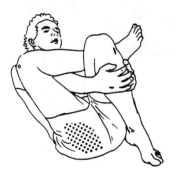

103 **Standing hamstring and buttock strengthening with resistance.** Bend at the waist and rest the elbows on a table. With a band around the ankles pull one leg behind. Control the leg as it returns to starting position and repeat slowly.

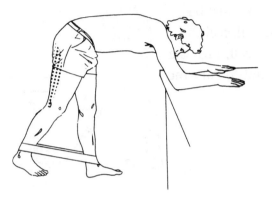

Calves

104 **Calf stretch.** Leaning against a wall, lift the arch of the foot slightly. Keep the hip and knee in a straight line and lean forward. Stretch each leg separately. Do not let the arch collapse to a flat-footed position as you do this stretch, as this may cause overstretched ligaments in the foot.

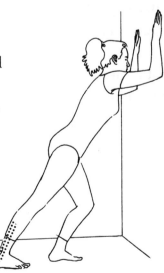

105 **Calf and toe flexor stretch.** With the toes and ankle bent back and resting against a step, keep the heel on the ground and lean forward. The back must be straight. You will feel the stretch on the calf; turn the foot in then out to vary the stretch.

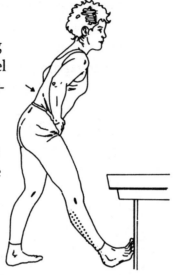

106 **Calf step stretch.** Standing on the edge of a step, slowly lower the heels over the edge of the step. Repeat with foot turned outwards, then inwards slightly, to stretch both heads of the calf muscle.

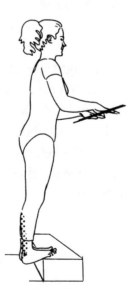

107 **Outer calf stretch.** Place a small object such as a crepe bandage under the arch of the foot. Keep the heel on the floor. Now lean forward, keeping the knee straight. Hold for 6–10 seconds, then bend the knee. If you get sore calves or Achilles tendons after sport, this exercise is ideal for you.

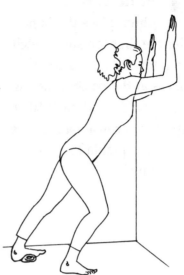

108 **Achilles stretch.** In the same leg position as exercise 104, bend the knee to stretch the Achilles tendon and soleus. This stretch can be made more effective by placing the toes against a step and bending them backwards (extension).

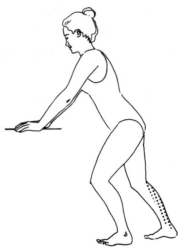

109 **Toe flexor stretch.**
While sitting, place the hand
under the first toe and stretch
it back towards the ankle.
Stiffness at the base of the big
toe (it should bend back 60–90
degrees) can cause pain in the
arch (called plantafascitis) or
'shin splints'.

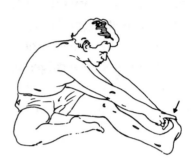

110 **Calf stretch and
strengthening (toe raises).** On
a step, let the ankle drop
below the step level. Feel the
stretch on the calf. Raise up on
the toes. Repeat with single leg
as well as both legs to
strengthen the calves and
ankles.

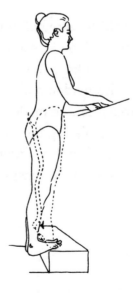

111 **Outer calf and thigh stretch.** While sitting, and with one leg bent, place the hand opposite the outstretched leg on the outside of the foot. Now pull the toes and ankle inwards as you straighten the knee.

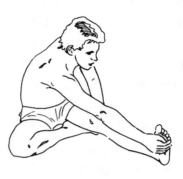

112 **Outer ankle strengthening.** Place an exercise band around the forefoot and pull the toes up and outwards. Keep the legs apart to be effective. An excellent exercise, combined with exercises 110, 111 and 113, if you have weak ankles, which you sprain or injure often.

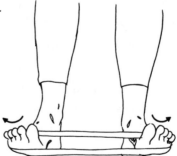

113 **Ankle strengthening and balance.** While standing, bend one leg. Go up on the toes and try to bend the knee directly over the foot. Do not let the arch of the foot collapse. You may need to hold on to something for balance, but only initially. To increase the difficulty of the exercise, close your eyes as you do it, or bounce a ball against a wall or on the ground while you are up on your toes.

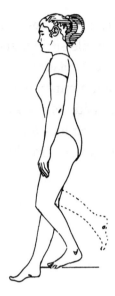

114 **Wobble board** — for improved balance. Use both feet initially, then progress to one foot and work the ankle in all directions. Try to hold on to something only minimally and if possible not at all. Using a few pillows on top of each other is ideal if you do not have access to a wobble board. When this feels too easy, try to do this with your eyes closed. Be careful though!

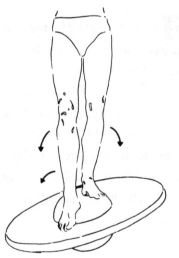

115 **Intrinsic foot strengthening.** While sitting, try to pick up pens or a towel to strengthen the intrinsic muscles of the foot. This is an ideal exercise if you have flat feet, as it strengthens the muscles that support the arch of the foot.

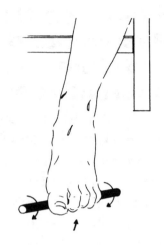

116 **Ankle mobility.** Clasp onto one foot and loosen the ankle by rotating the foot in circles one way, then the other. Then loosen the bones in the forefoot with your hand by flexing and extending them. This is an ideal exercise if your feet are tired at the end of a working day.

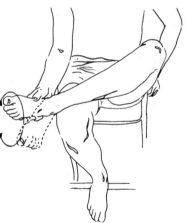

Exercises Not Recommended and Safe Alternatives

Any exercise performed at high speed with lack of control can create instability around a joint and musculo-skeletal problems may develop. Always work at a controlled pace with good form when you are exercising. Consult a sports specialist if a particular exercise causes pain. An exercise may cause discomfort but it should not cause pain!

The following exercises are not recommended as they can be potentially harmful, particularly when performed at high speed or with high repetitions. Safe alternatives are suggested. If you are training at an elite level, some of these exercises may be appropriate, but consult with a sports specialist first if you are unsure.

117 **Double straight-leg raise** — incorrect. Performing the double straight-leg raises with the back arched is stressful for the lower back, because the hip flexor (or iliopsoas) is worked in a shortened range when there is not sufficient strength in the abdominals. This can stress the lower back.

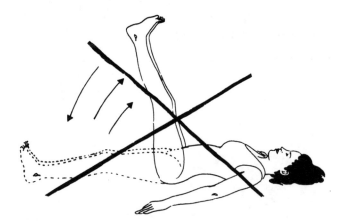

118 **Inner-range leg cycling** — correct. As an alternative to exercise 117, work only in the range where you can maintain a flat back. Working between 45 and 90 degrees from the floor is acceptable if the back can be maintained flat on the floor. Bracing the abdominals will prevent arching of the back.

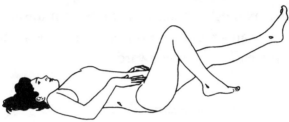

119 **Hip hyperextension** — incorrect. Hip hyperextension, often performed in aerobics classes at high speed, with no control, is potentially stressful to the lower back — the ligaments, muscles and discs.

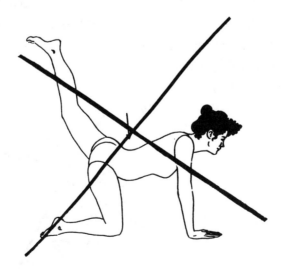

120 **Buttock strengthening** — correct. As an alternative to exercise 119, control the movement by flexing the foot and resting down on the elbows. Keeping the buttocks tight also reduces stress on the back. Do not move greater than 10 degrees beyond the horizontal plane. Using a bent leg to perform this exercise is another way to strengthen the buttocks (or gluteus maximus). Do not let the foot turn inwards or outwards, as this can stress the lower back or hip joint area, and do not let the back drop downwards.

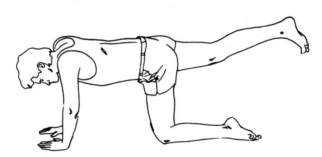

121 **Straight-leg and jack-knife sit-ups** — incorrect. Performed at high speed with high repetitions, these exercises can be potentially stressful on the lower back, because they result in tightened hip flexors. While jack-knife sit-ups should never be done, straight-leg sit-ups are permissible if performed in a controlled manner, not at speed.

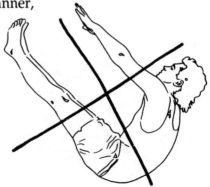

122 **Bent-leg sit-ups** — correct. These sit-ups are a safe alternative to the sit-ups in exercise 121. Exercises 71–79 show how to isolate and strengthen both the upper and lower segments of the abdominals, effectively and safely.

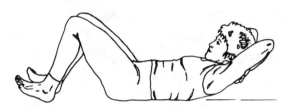

123 **Hurdler's stretch** — incorrect. This is where one leg is outstretched and the other is bent at the knee and turned backwards. There is potential damage to the inner structures of the knee, in this position. To stretch the hamstrings and lower back, always turn the knee outwards with the foot resting on the inside of the outstretched leg.

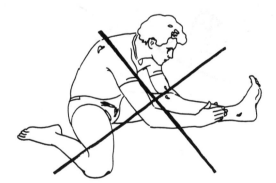

124 **Hamstring stretch** — correct. With one foot on the inside of the thigh of the outstretched leg, place hands on either side of it. Gently try to bend the elbows and ease forward. Do not just curve the head and shoulders forward. Keep the back straight.

125 **Back hyperextension** — incorrect. Raising the legs and arms at the same time places unnecessary stress on the lower back. Working the arms then the legs, either independently or oppositely, is less stressful.

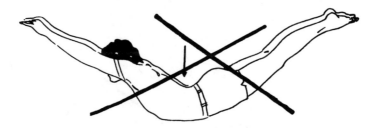

126 **Opposite arm and leg** — correct. Stretch them out long, rather than arching too far. Repeat both sides. (Refer to exercise 56.)

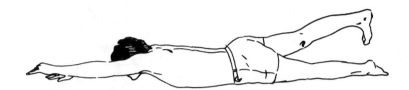

127 **Touching the toes and sustained forward flexion** — bouncing while touching the toes — incorrect. Sustained forward flexion is a position often used in fitness classes. However, it overloads the discs in the lumbar spine. It should only be used as a stretch, if at all, not as a position for working the arms. Touching the toes and bouncing to get further should never be attempted.

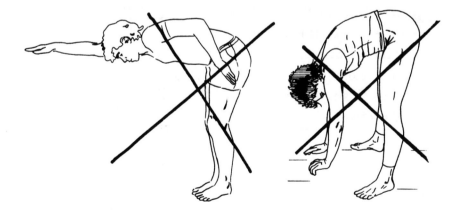

128 **Circular neck rotations** — incorrect. Rotating the neck through a full circle one way then the other can close down some of the joints in the cervical spine and impinge on the nerve structures. Exercises 1–6 show how to exercise the neck correctly and safely.

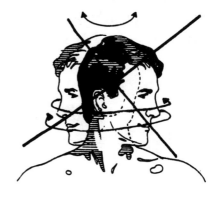

129 **Full squats** — incorrect. Bouncing while in a full-squat position with the buttocks close to the floor is very stressful for the knees.

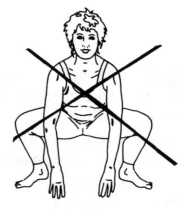

130 **Modified squat position** — correct. It is safe to exercise the quadriceps if the knee is not taken greater than 90 degrees. This is least stressful for the knee.

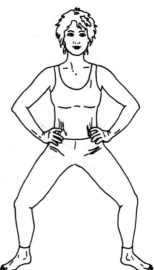

8
Daily Routines

This chapter shows exercises suitable for daily muscle maintenance. These routines will not improve your cardiovascular fitness, but they will improve your general flexibility and strength. You should notice an improvement in your posture, especially if you are doing the routines in addition to your regular aerobic exercise, and you will certainly feel freer in your movements while playing sport.

To improve your flexibility, you must take your muscles to greater than their normal range (i.e. overload them) regularly. They should be taken to a point of slight discomfort, but not to the point of pain. In time the muscles adapt to this regular overloading and become longer. To achieve this, you will have to stretch for a minimum of three times per week, but an optimum flexibility regime is stretching for 10–15 minutes daily. The maximum number of repetitions of the routines is twice daily, for 15–20 minutes. It is particularly important to include stretching in both the warm-up and cool-down of your sport or activity.

Try not to stretch when you are cold and have not loosened up at all. In other words, it is better to stretch in the evening, when your muscles and joints are a little looser, than first thing in the morning.

If you have not exercised for some time and have taken all the precautionary measures outlined in Chapter 4, commence with level 1. When you find these exercises too easy, progress to level 2, then to level 3. If you currently exercise regularly, practise level 1, but you should be able to move to level 2 and 3 quite quickly.

Hold all stretches for a minimum of 6–10 seconds—the longer you hold a stretch, the more effective it will be—and repeat mobility exercises four to five times. Commence strengthening exercises with six to eight repetitions, then progress to eight to twelve. When this becomes too easy, rest, then complete another set, incorporating the same number of repetitions. Always think of the muscle you are working, and aim for quality movements rather than quantity.

Level 1 — Beginners

Preparing for your routine

Circle your arms forwards and backwards eight to ten times. Repeat. While standing, hug one knee up to your chest, then the other. Use a stationary bicycle or mini-trampoline to work out on for 10–12 minutes. Going for a brisk walk will also prepare you for the following exercises.

Mobility exercises and stretches

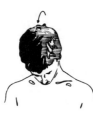

1. Neck flexion (× 1)

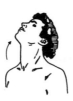

2. Neck extension (× 1)

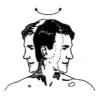

3. Neck rotation (× 1)

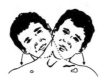

4. Neck side flexion (× 1)

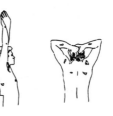

19. Mid-back and shoulder mobility exercise

24. Outside shoulder stretch

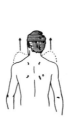

26. Shoulder shrugs

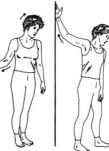
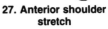

27. Anterior shoulder stretch

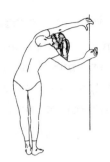

37. Side trunk and hip stretch

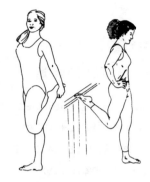

84. Quadriceps stretch

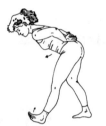

92. Hamstring stretch: standing

49. Knee hug stretch

41. Cat stretch: extension

42. Cat stretch: flexion

43. Lower back release

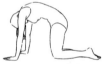

45. Passive back arch and abdominal stretch

46. Gentle back release

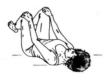

47. Spinal release stretch

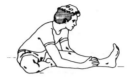

96. Hamstring and lower back

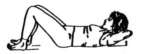

**50. Spinal rotation
stretch: lying**

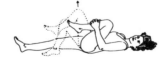

**48. Pelvis and lower
back release**

Strengthening exercises

71. Sit-ups: beginners

**75. Beginners' lower abdominals
strengthening**

80. Inner thigh stretch and oblique strengthening

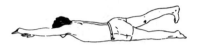

56. Opposite leg and arm lift strengthening

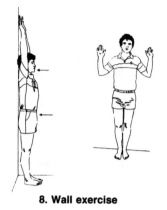

8. Wall exercise

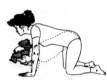

67. Hip strengthening

13. Pectoral and tricep strengthening

Level 2— Intermediate

Preparing for your routine

Loosen up the arms with large circular movements. Try incorporating a light jog, a brisk walk, skipping or cycling into your preparation for the exercises. Include these exercises in your daily regime if you are already engaged in a fitness program. Many of these exercises are in the beginners' regime but the new exercises included will provide a challenge.

Mobility exercises and stretches

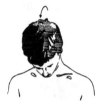

1. Neck flexion

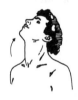

2. Neck extension

3. Neck rotation

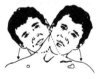

4. Neck side flexion

5. Neck stretch

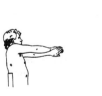

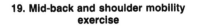

19. Mid-back and shoulder mobility exercise

24. Outside shoulder stretch

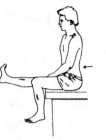

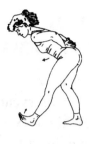

25. Shoulder rotations: sitting or standing

91. Hamstring stretch: sitting

92. Hamstring stretch: standing

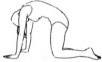

41. Cat stretch: extension

42. Cat stretch: flexion

11. Pectoral stretch

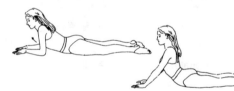

45. Passive back arch and abdominal stretch

20. Shoulder mobility

21. Shoulder and mid-back stretch

50. Spinal rotation stretch: lying

102. Upper hamstring stretch: lying

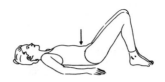

46. Lower back release: knees to chest

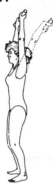

18. Mid-back spine and
shoulder mobility: using
a rod or towel

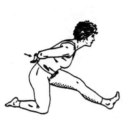

95. Hamstring stretch:
kneeling

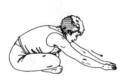

64. Posterior hip stretch

Strengthening exercises

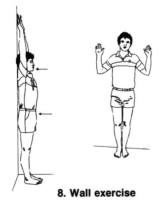

8. Wall exercise

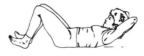

72. Sit-ups: intermediate

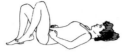

76. Intermediate lower abdominals strengthening

67. Hip strengthening

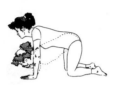

13. Pectoral and tricep strengthening

14. Shoulder girdle strengthening

77. Advanced lower abdominals strengthening

Level 3— Advanced

Preparing for your routine

Jogging, brisk walking, cycling or skipping for 15–30 minutes prior to trying the following exercises is recommended. The exercises in this section are only suitable if you have completed levels 1 and 2 easily, or if you currently do regular aerobic exercise.

Mobility exercises and stretches

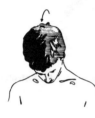
1. Neck flexion

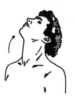
2. Neck extension

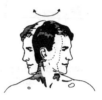
3. Neck rotation

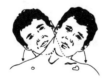
4. Neck side flexion

5. Neck stretch

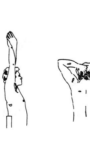
19. Mid-back and shoulder mobility exercise

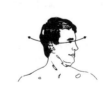
18. Mid-back spine and shoulder mobility: using a rod or towel

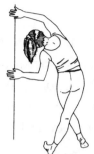

38. Side trunk, shoulder and hip stretch

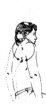

25. Shoulder rotations: sitting or standing

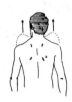

26. Shoulder shrugs

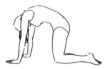

40. Advanced shoulder and mid-back stretch

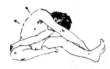

36. Side trunk and shoulder stretch

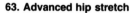

10. Advanced neck and upper back strengthening

41. Cat stretch: extension

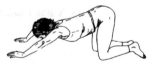

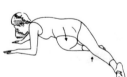

42. Cat stretch: flexion

63. Advanced hip stretch

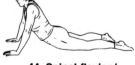

44. Spinal flexion/ extension stretch

20. Shoulder mobility

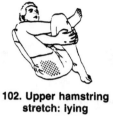

102. Upper hamstring
stretch: lying

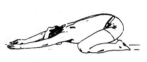

43. Lower back release

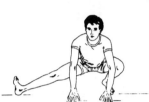

81. Inner thigh stretch:
standing/squatting

Strengthening exercises

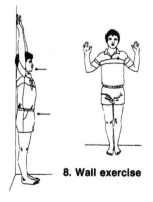

8. Wall exercise

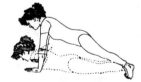

15. Full push-up

56. Opposite leg and arm lift
strengthening

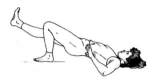

70. Buttock and upper hamstring advanced

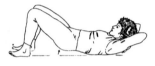

67. Hip strengthening

72. Sit-ups: intermediate

73. Sit-ups: advanced

76. Intermediate lower abdominals strengthening

77. Advanced lower abdominals strengthening

9
Special Groups

This chapter outlines daily routines for specific groups that are most vulnerable to developing poor posture and therefore muscle-related problems. Each section will provide you with an easy-to-follow regime that you can incorporate into your work situation or daily exercise routine, whichever is convenient.

Holding the body in one position for extended periods of time leads to stiff and sore muscles and joints, particularly of the neck and back. The desk/computer workers', travelers' and musicians' routines are all designed to relieve this problem. Try to take a break from your sedentary position and do the exercises throughout the day, every hour if possible.

For the over-fifties, a general stretching program is shown, while for new mothers, easy-to-do exercises are provided. For sportspeople, some general stretches are outlined.

A special section for healthy back care is included, but be sure to check with your physical therapist before following this routine.

Desk/ Computer Workers

When you are restricted to sitting for extended periods of time, the body can become very stiff in its muscles and joints. The following exercises can minimize this effect. Practice them whenever possible as a break from your desk work.

Try to keep the body moving as much as possible within the confined space, and use a back support or a small towel rolled up and placed in the small of your back to support your back when sitting. Take breaks from your desk at a minimum of every half an hour for 5–8 minutes, especially if you are working on a computer or typing. Go for a walk in your breaks, if possible.

Exercises

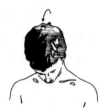

1. Neck flexion

2. Neck extension

3. Neck rotation

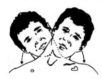

4. Neck side flexion

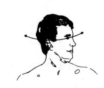

5. Neck stretch

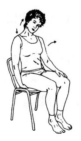

6. Sitting neck stretch

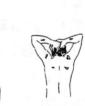

19. Mid-back and shoulder mobility exercise

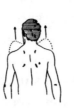
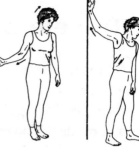

25. Shoulder rotations: sitting or standing

26. Shoulder shrugs

27. Anterior shoulder stretch

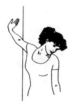
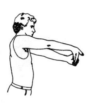
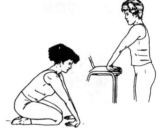

28. Fingers, wrist, shoulder and neck stretch

29. Wrist and finger stretch

30. Forearm flexor stretch

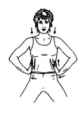
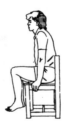
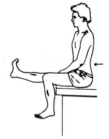

31. Hands on hips

17. Sitting pectoral and shoulder strengthening

91. Hamstring stretch: sitting

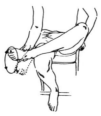

116. Ankle mobility

Travelers

Whether you travel by air or drive long distances, traveling can be very stressful for the body. The following exercises can be done, either while sitting or when you take a break from driving. For plane travel, go for regular walks to stretch the legs on longer trips, and do the following exercises every hour or so while you are seated. For the driver, always use a rolled-up towel in the lower back if you are on the road for extended periods, and have a rest from driving and do some stretches every 2–3 hours.

Exercises

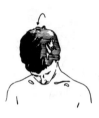

1. Neck flexion

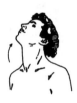

2. Neck extension

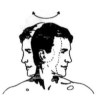

3. Neck rotation

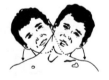

4. Neck side flexion

5. Neck stretch

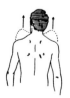

26. Shoulder shrugs

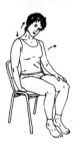

6. Sitting neck stretch

Do the following stretches when taking a break from driving.

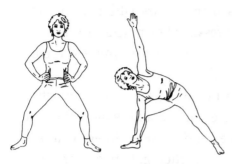

23. Advanced mid-back stretch

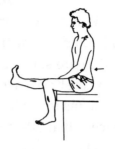

91. Hamstring stretch: sitting

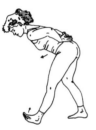

92. Hamstring stretch: standing

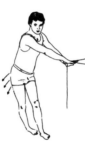

66. Outer hip stretch

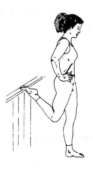

84. Quadriceps stretch

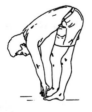

100. Inner and outer hamstring stretch

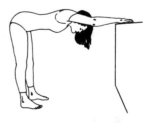

39. Advanced mid-back spine mobility

Musicians

Playing a musical instrument usually requires many hours sitting in a fixed position. Whether you are a professional or practise for leisure, you will benefit from these exercises. Even if you are a conductor, they are suitable.

Try to take breaks whenever possible when you are practicing, and do the following exercises. Spend a little more time on the stretches that affect the areas and muscles where you feel stiffness when you are playing or practicing. Between practice or performance sessions, the stretches and strengthening exercises shown in the healthy back care section would also be highly recommended.

Exercises

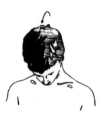

1. Neck flexion

2. Neck extension

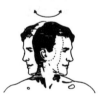

3. Neck rotation

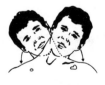

4. Neck side flexion

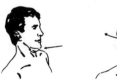

5. Neck stretch

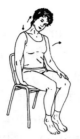

6. Sitting neck stretch

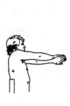

19. Mid-back and shoulder mobility exercise

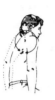

25. Shoulder rotations: sitting or standing

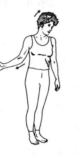

27. Anterior shoulder stretch

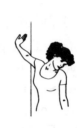

28. Fingers, wrist, shoulder and neck stretch

29. Wrist and finger stretch

30. Forearm flexor stretch

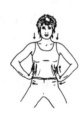

31. Hands on hips

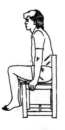

17. Sitting pectoral and shoulder strengthening

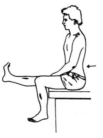

91. Hamstring stretch: sitting

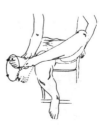

116. Ankle mobility

The Over-fifties

No matter what your age, it is never too late to get a little fitter. Be gentle on your body when you do these exercises; push to discomfort but not through pain. If you are uncertain whether any of the exercises are harmful to you, check with your physical therapist. Work within your limits, but take all the stretches through the full range, and try to do them at least once a day. Perform them on a carpeted floor, not a soft bed.

If you have arthritis, aquarobics classes, swimming or brisk walking will help you to maintain cardiovascular fitness and keep your muscles supple and strong. Pain from arthritis can be markedly reduced if you keep fit. Arthritis itself is usually the result of inactivity, and far less often the result of excessive activity. Exercising regularly will improve circulation through the body, and keeping flexible and strong will reduce the stress taken by the affected joints.

Always combine these exercises with your regular aerobic activity. When you are warmer, you will be able to stretch a little more easily. Going for a 15–20 minute walk or bicycle ride, or just circling the arms, both forwards and backwards, eight to ten times each way, will loosen the muscles. Next try to hug each knee onto the chest, while standing, if possible. Also while standing, bend the knees slightly and rotate them each way. Loosen the ankles and feet by rotating them with your hands while you are sitting.

Exercises

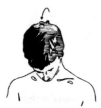 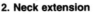 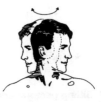

1. Neck flexion   2. Neck extension   3. Neck rotation

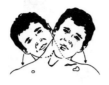

4. Neck side flexion

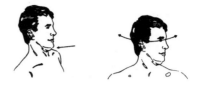

5. Neck stretch

24. Outside shoulder stretch

25. Shoulder rotations: sitting or standing

32. Posterior shoulder stretch

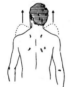

26. Shoulder shrugs

28. Fingers, wrist, shoulder and neck stretch

86. Hip mobility

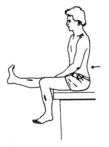

91. Hamstring stretch: sitting —
progress to 96

41. Cat stretch: extension

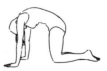

42. Cat stretch: flexion

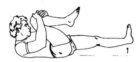

43. Lower back release

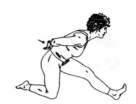

45. Passive back arch and abdominal stretch

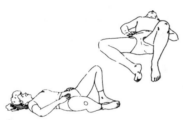

49. Knee hug stretch

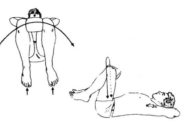

52. Double leg spinal rotation

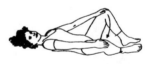

80. Inner thigh stretch and oblique strengthening

48. Pelvis and lower back release

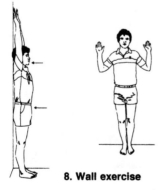

8. Wall exercise

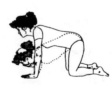

13. Pectoral and tricep strengthening

54. Back-strengthening single leg lift

55. Back-strengthening single arm lift

56. Opposite leg and arm lift strengthening

68. Outer hip strengthening

67. Hip strengthening

75. Beginners' lower abdominals strengthening

Finish your exercise routine with exercise 43, lower back release.

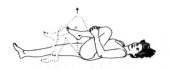

43. Lower back release

New Mothers

So often women hurt themselves or experience neck or back ache, previously unknown to them, once they have a child. Finding the time to look after yourself when you are a new mother is indeed a challenge, but, for the short time it takes to do a few general exercises, the results will be rewarding. Try to recommence your aerobic routine as soon as possible (with your doctor's approval), to ensure your body regains its prenatal fitness in the shortest possible time.

Focus on keeping the shoulders, neck and mid-back flexible and strong (particularly if you are breastfeeding), and strengthening the muscles of the pelvis and abdomen (as soon as Nature permits). Your physical therapist can advise you of specific pelvic floor exercises, while the following exercises will work on the other important areas. Take care with all exercises and progress to the advanced daily routines when the following are too easy.

Exercises
Neck and shoulders

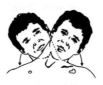

4. Neck side flexion

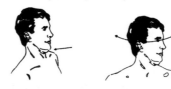

5. Neck stretch

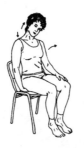

6. Sitting neck stretch

7. Sitting neck and shoulder stretch

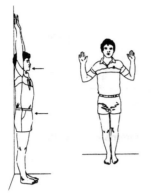

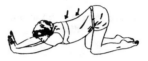

9. Neck and upper back strengthening

8. Wall exercise

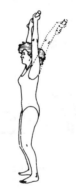

11. Pectoral stretch

13. Pectoral and tricep strengthening

18. Mid-back spine and shoulder mobility: using a rod or towel

Spine and hips

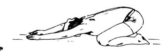

41. Cat stretch: extension   **42. Cat stretch: flexion**   **43. Lower back release**

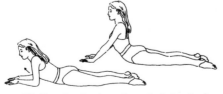

45. Passive back arch and abdominal stretch

46. Gentle back release

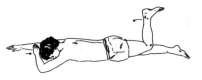

56. Opposite leg and arm lift strengthening

57. Alternate swimming

Abdominals

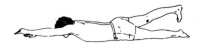

71. Sit-ups: beginners

72. Sit-ups: intermediate

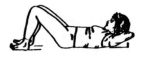

74. Oblique strengthening

75. Beginners' lower abdominals strengthening

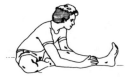

96. Hamstring and lower back

Sportspeople and Athletes

If you participate in social sport, it is very important to warm up and stretch a little prior to your activity to minimize your risk of injury. Whether you jog, play tennis, squash, cricket or lawn bowls, or go for a regular walk, the following stretches are highly recommended. Include them in your general warm-up period.

Warm-up

Often walking to the venue where you are to play your sport is sufficient warm-up. Going for a 5 minute jog on an oval next to the tennis court may also be possible. For the stretches, identify which are most appropriate for your sport: for example, for swimming, focus on the shoulders and spine; and for jogging, concentrate on the legs and lower back. However, also include exercises for the muscles that you do not use in your sport in your daily muscle maintenance routine, to achieve muscle balance.

Exercises

The following general stretches are suitable for all sports:

Neck and shoulders

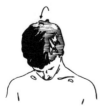   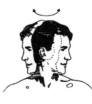

1. Neck flexion   2. Neck extension   3. Neck rotation

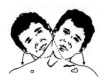
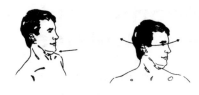

4. Neck side flexion

5. Neck stretch

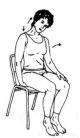

6. Sitting neck stretch

11. Pectoral stretch

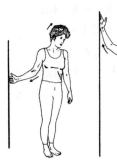
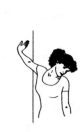

27. Anterior shoulder stretch

28. Fingers, wrist, shoulder and neck stretch

24. Outside shoulder stretch

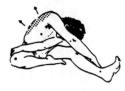

36. Side trunk and shoulder stretch

Spine and hips

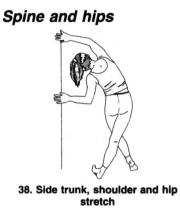

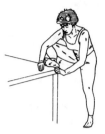

38. Side trunk, shoulder and hip stretch

101. Outer hip stretch

Hamstrings and calves

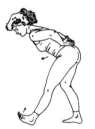

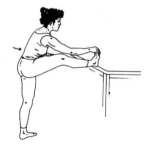

92. Hamstring stretch: standing

94. Hamstring stretch: using a fence or table

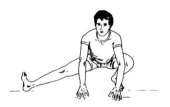

98. Combined hamstring and inner thigh stretch

Quadriceps

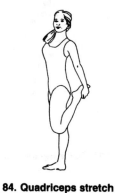

84. Quadriceps stretch

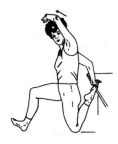

87. Hip flexor stretch: kneeling

Calves

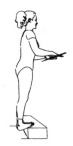

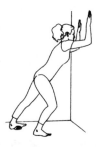

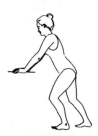

106. Calf step stretch   107. Outer calf stretch   108. Achilles stretch

109. Toe flexor stretch

A Fit Back

A fit and healthy back is one that is strong, flexible and capable of withstanding the many stresses to which it is subjected every day. Whether we are sitting or playing sport, the lower back is subject to stress and to loads far in excess of our own body weight. The majority of back aches are muscular in origin, and could possibly have been prevented if the individual had been more flexible and a little stronger in the muscles that support the back, and had maintained better posture.

There are several key reasons people hurt their back: poor lifting technique; sitting in one position for too long without a break; and general lack of aerobic and/or muscle fitness. To achieve a fitter back through exercise, you will need to focus on stretching the hamstrings, hip flexors, and back and neck extensors, and strengthening the abdominals, quadriceps and shoulder/back muscles (e.g. the latissimus dorsi).

The following routine should be performed daily to be effective, but consult with your physical therapist if you currently experience back pain to find out if the exercises are suitable for your specific complaint.

Exercises

Beginners

49. Knee hug stretch

97. Lying hamstring stretch

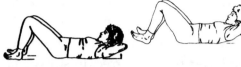

71. Sit-ups: beginners   **72. Sit-ups: intermediate**   **75. Beginners' lower abdominals strengthening**

76. Intermediate lower abdominals strengthening   **74. Oblique strengthening**

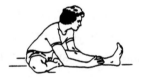

59. Lower back stretch   **56. Opposite leg and arm lift strengthening**

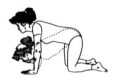

13. Pectoral and tricep strengthening   **41. Cat stretch: extension**

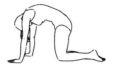

42. Cat stretch: flexion

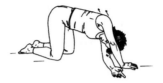

21. Shoulder and mid-back stretch

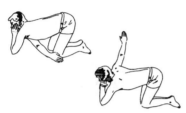

22. Shoulder and mid-back mobility

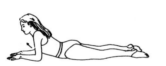

43. Lower back release

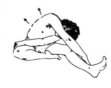

45. Passive back arch and abdominal stretch

Intermediate

Add in these exercises when you feel the beginners' exercises are becoming too easy.

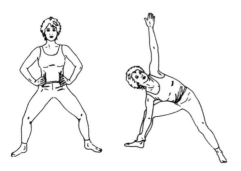

23. Advanced mid-back stretch

36. Side trunk and hip stretch

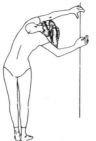
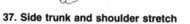
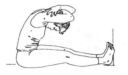

37. Side trunk and shoulder stretch

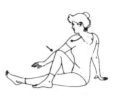

53. Spinal rotation stretch: sitting

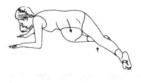

60. Advanced spinal stretch

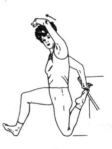

63. Advanced hip stretch

67. Hip strengthening

87. Hip flexor stretch: kneeling

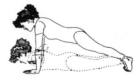

15. Full push-up

Advanced

Add these exercises to the above routine.

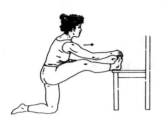

99. Advanced hamstring and calf stretch

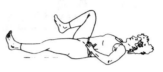

77. Advanced lower abdominals strengthening

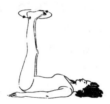

78. Athletes' lower abdominals strengthening

Finish with exercise 50, spinal rotation stretch: lying, and exercise 43, lower back release.

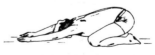

50. Spinal rotation stretch: lying   **43. Lower back release**

10
Muscle Care

When you have sore muscles or pain, deciding whether to rest, exercise, consult a specialist or listen to a friend's advice can be a dilemma. This chapter outlines self-help measures for when you injure your muscles, and the pros and cons of various methods of treatment. First, though, we need to clarify some of the common terms used in relation to muscle care.

Muscle Injury Terminology

Trauma This word is used interchangeably with 'injury'. A direct trauma is an injury produced by a direct impact to an area. An indirect trauma is produced when a soft tissue (muscle, tendon or ligament) is injured or damaged without impact to the area, for instance, a muscle strain.

Acute This refers to an injury that occurred recently, usually during the last 2–3 days.

Chronic This refers to an injury that has been present in the body for more than a few weeks.

Hematoma A bruise.

Contusion This refers to a bruise that has started to collect or consolidate in an area. A contusion can happen with a corked thigh, for example.

Muscle strain This refers to a tear of some of the myofibrils of the muscle. Repetitive stress over a period of time on a specific area may cause microtrauma (or small repetitive tears) to any part of a muscle or its tendon (e.g. a chronic hamstring strain). A macrotrauma refers to one specific injury to an area (such as a corked thigh). Muscle strains are usually classified as first, second or third degree, depending on the severity of the injury. Muscle strains that take 2–10 days to heal are usually said to be first-degree strains. A third-degree strain describes a ruptured muscle. Depending on where the latter occurs, the muscle often heals in a new bunched-up and shortened position, resulting in surrounding muscles doing the work it used to do.

Muscle soreness This refers to the stiffness that occurs after doing unfamiliar or excessive exercise. It usually does not occur until 24 hours after the activity, and is relieved by massage or gentle stretching.

Ligament sprain This occurs when a ligament is overstretched. It is again classified as a first- to third-degree sprain. A first degree is a partial tear of some of the fibres of the ligament (e.g. a sprained ankle) and takes 4–6 weeks to totally repair itself, although with taping for support, return to sport is usually possible earlier than this. A third-degree sprain refers to a ruptured ligament. This is common in the knee, and requires surgical repair within 7–10 days following the injury in many instances. Conservative treatment, meaning strengthening exercises and physiotherapeutic modalities, may sometimes be used, depending on which ligament is ruptured, how actively the person is engaged in sport and so on.

Musculoligamentous injury This occurs when both the muscle and the ligament are damaged in an area. It is common in the neck or back after a car accident or when injury occurs from heavy lifting.

Tendonitis 'Itis' refers to inflammation, so 'tendonitis' refers to inflammation of a tendon. Most tendons are enclosed within a sheath and the tendon becomes inflamed within the sheath with repetitive stress or abnormal loading. Shoulder tendonitis is common if imbalance of muscles exists around the shoulder, causing impingement of tendons such as the biceps or other shoulder muscles.

Bursitis This is inflammation of the bursa, which is a fluid-filled sac made of connective tissue that lies between bone and tendon to prevent friction occurring with movement. It becomes inflamed with abnormal loading (due to muscle imbalance) or through overexercising a specific area.

Capsulitis This refers to inflammation of the capsule that surrounds a synovial joint. It is most common in the shoulder.

The RICE(D) Principle

The immediate action to take when acute trauma occurs is to use ice in accordance with the Rice(D) principle. This is outlined below:

R = Rest Be sure to take the load or weight off the injured area. If exercising is painful, do not continue.

I = Ice Apply ice as soon as possible. This can be done by wrapping fresh ice in a damp towel, using a commercially made icepack or a bag of frozen peas, or by filling a paper cup with water and freezing it, then massaging it on the affected area. An icepack is the preferred alternative. It should stay on for 10–15 minutes — no longer!

C = **Compression** Apply a compression (stretch) bandage to the area to prevent excessive swelling. Do not use non-elastic tape.

E = **Elevation** Try to keep the injured area elevated to permit gravity to assist reduction of swelling.

D = **Diagnosis** Consult a doctor, physical therapist or other specialist if pain and swelling do not settle within 24 hours, to receive a professional diagnosis and advice regarding your complaint.

Ice Versus Heat Treatment

When we traumatize soft tissue, bleeding occurs in the area. If the muscle fibers are damaged, the normal physiological muscle pump that assists the movement of blood from peripheral areas to more central regions in impeded, and swelling from a traumatized area is not effectively removed. Ice has a local effect of closing down blood vessels (vasoconstriction), which prevents excessive bleeding. The hypothalamus of the brain responds to this local vasoconstriction by sending blood to the deeper vessels to counteract this effect. Mild vasodilation (opening up of blood vessels) occurs, and this extra flow deep to the area assists to reduce swelling as more fluid is pumped back to the heart. Vasoconstriction then recurs, causing a mild pumping effect in the soft tissue. All this takes place in 10–15 minutes.

Use caution when applying ice to neck and shoulder area as prolonged exposure can damage nerves. Consult a doctor.

For an acutely sprained ankle an ice bucket may be used. This consists of ice cubes in water. Immerse the swollen limb and when it is numb, take it out and start flexing and extending the foot. Repeat for 10–15 minutes every 2 hours, maybe three or four times, and the severe swelling will usually subside.

In an acute injury, while there is any sign of bleeding, heat should not be used as it causes vasodilation, which increases the bleeding. For most sprains it is fine to use heat after 72 hours. However, for acute traumas such as partially torn hamstrings, where bruising is present in the entire muscle belly, until yellowing of the bruise begins to show, indicating healing, do *not* use heat! In this instance (as well as in the case of a corked thigh) ice may need to be used for up to a week — even longer.

Ointments and Rubs

There is a lack of scientific research to support the effectiveness of many of the lubricants currently available on the market. However, if we analyze most of these products and their pharmacological contents, their role seems less questionable. Most heat rubs contain the substance methyl salicylate, a derivative of ethyl salicylate, which forms the basis of aspirin. (Interestingly, methyl salicylate is also the commercial name for wintergreen oil, a centuries-old remedy for use on muscle aches and pains.) Aspirin is used to reduce inflammation, and provides a mild analgesic effect; so maybe heat rubs do assist with reducing the inflammation caused by trauma.

Heat rubs also cause a counterirritant effect on the skin. This creates a superficial chemical reaction, giving rise to redness and warmth in the skin locally and a subsequent increased blood flow to the area. This local response is claimed to assist with circulation deeper to the area, although to what extent is as yet unknown.

Most people use heat rubs because of their mild analgesic effect and because of the warmth produced in the area to which they are applied. Heat rubs may be used both before and after sport. The rubs should not replace warm-up and stretches but, used on a painful area and combined with massage, can provide considerable relief from mild muscular aches or pains, particularly post-exercise muscle soreness. It is safe to apply these rubs several times each day.

Never use heat rubs on the face, under the arm or in the groin area.

Commonly Asked Questions

Should I exercise if I have a cold or viral infection?

When your body is carrying some form of infection, the best way to assist it to fight the infection and promote the healing process is to sleep or rest whenever possible. If you have a temperature, rest is even more important. Colds tend to afflict us more when we are run down physically — maybe you were overtraining? — therefore, you may need to re-evaluate your fitness program (or lifestyle). Viral infections often affect the nervous system, so if you exercise you may feel worse afterwards. Let your body have a few days' rest if you are feeling tired or run down, or if you have an infection in your body. When you do return to your sport or activity, it will be much more enjoyable and less stressful.

Will supports that keep an area warm help my injury?

There are many supports available, which are not guards to protect an area, but when worn keep an area warm. The physiological mechanism of how these supports work is difficult to explain. It seems some type of counterirritant effect is again provided, improving blood supply to the area. For chronic muscle stiffness and strains past their acute phase, many athletes find these supports helpful for keeping an area warm. Providing accurate diagnosis has eliminated a major problem, and the causes of an injury have been ascertained, the use of these supports to maintain warmth in an area is recommended.

Corked thighs and tight hamstrings are examples of injuries where these supports may be of benefit.

When I have sore muscles after exercise, should I rest or continue with exercise?

By stretching prior to and at the completion of your sport, it is possible to reduce post-exercise soreness. Massage will also reduce muscle soreness. However, if you have stiff, sore muscles from doing unfamiliar or excessive exercise, it is best to stretch and do a lighter or different form of exercise. Rest will only tighten your muscles further.

Why do I get stitches and cramps when I run?

There are few scientific reasons for stitches in the abdomen and anterior shoulder, or cramps in the abdomen or lower limb. Prior to the 1980s, it was thought that cramps were due to a lack of salt in the body, but this hypothesis has since been dispelled, as our Western diet provides adequate levels of sodium (salt).

The current explanation for cramps is dehydration, or inadequate fluid in the body prior to exercising. Before any vigorous exercise session, an increase in fluid intake (two to three glasses of water) is recommended. Do not drink strong salt-based drinks as these will have a counterproductive effect. Weak drinks of this nature are not a problem.

Another theory for abdominal cramps is that they are caused by milk-based products, which are very slow to digest, taken too soon before an exercise session. You will need to minimize the intake of these types of food before exercise to know if this is what is causing the cramping.

In the case of stitches, clinical findings outweigh any scientific theory. In the author's clinical experience, a small section

of fibritic tissue or a muscle spasm in the diaphragm or iliopsoas (hip flexor) muscle is often found when the technique of
deep connective tissue massage is used in the abdominal region.
This method may free the scar tissue or muscle spasm and usually the stitches do not return, unless some other biomechanical
reason exists. A tight and shortened iliopsoas or fibrous tissue
of the abdominal muscle postnatally is often a common precursor to stitches.

Stitches of the shoulder are not so clearly understood. It is
of clinical interest that athletes complaining of shoulder stitches
are usually round-shouldered, have a curved-forward mid-back
spine and tight pectoral muscles. This type of posture severely
overloads the mid-back and upper back. Nerves from this
region refer to the anterior chest wall, so it does seem that
shoulder stitches are the result of referred pain. With postural
corrective exercises, mobilization of the spine and stretching of
pectorals, the problem is usually relieved.

How do I know when I can return to full sporting activity, and what precautions can I take to prevent trauma recurring?

If you were badly injured, your specialist or therapist is the
person to answer this question but if you have been treating
yourself, the following points may help you decide:

- Be sure not to return to sport too soon following trauma.
  An area is healing long after the pain has disappeared.
- Ligaments take 2–6 weeks to heal completely.
- Mild muscle strains take 2–14 days to heal, but more severe
  strains can take 3–6 weeks.
- Cartilage trauma takes 3–6 weeks and, if torn, may need to
  be operated on (this applies especially to a torn cartilage in
  the knee). Procedures such as arthroscopy permit rapid

recovery and return to sport if the ligament of the knee is not damaged as well.

• Bone fractures take 2–3 months or longer to heal.

• Stress fractures take a minimum of 4–6 weeks to heal sufficiently for full weight-bearing activities to resume.

• Tendonitis, musculoligamentous strains and contusions (from direct trauma impact) are variable in how long they take to heal. The healing time is dependent on the acuteness, extent and mechanism of the injury, and the time that the area has been traumatized prior to treatment. Overuse injuries may need considerable rest or a change in training methods, as compared with acute injuries, where all treatment is aimed at return to sport as soon as it is safe to do so.

• Children's muscle and tendon injuries heal more quickly than adults', but if damage to the bony growth plates has occurred (such as in the knee), rest from sports may be needed for 2–3 months. Seeking advice in the early stages, when a child complains of pain, can prevent these problems.

The following precautions should be taken to minimize the risk of recurrence of a problem:

• Use taping or a guard to support the injured area.

• Try to identify the demands and skills of the sport to which you are returning. Consider your current level of fitness; is it adequate? If you have had to rest due to injury, you must regain flexibility and strength in the injured area, in addition to your pre-injury fitness level. Does your sport require agility skills, flexibility or specific strength (see p. 38)? Reassess technique regularly and play practice matches prior to competition sport. Consult a sports specialist for further advice regarding your training programme if you are returning to sport from having an overuse problem.

Checklist

✔ Self-help for soft tissue trauma is to use the RICE(D) principle — R = Rest, I = Ice, C = Compression, E = Elevation, D = Diagnosis.

✔ If the problem does not settle or show signs of improvement within 24–48 hours post-injury, consult a specialist.

✔ For long-term care of an injury, do not return too soon to sport and prepare your body in all aspects of your sport prior to returning to play.

While you are injured, try to participate in some other form of exercise to retain your aerobic fitness level. If you cannot run, swim. If you cannot swim, cycle. If you cannot cycle, walk. If you are unable to undertake any of these activities because of pain, you can still stretch regularly to maintain muscle flexibility and tone.

The Final Word
on Muscles

Do you feel you understand your body a little better now? I hope you are enjoying doing your daily fitness regime. Remember, it will be difficult when you start, but with perseverance the routine will become easier and a part of your daily life.

Hopefully, *Stretching for Flexibility and Health* has dispelled the myth that lack of fitness is a natural part of growing old. No matter what your age, you can always improve your muscle fitness. Regular stretching and strengthening, keeping aerobically fit and sound nutrition are the keys to good health. As you become fitter, you will have much more energy to carry out your daily chores. Once you are fully involved in your fitness program, you will wonder how you ever lived without it. Furthermore, no matter what level or type of sport you play, you will be pleasantly surprised at the extra ease with which you are able to play it, when you incorporate some of the exercises described in this book, either as part of your warm-up or cool-down, or as part of a daily regime.

If you do not currently engage in regular sport of exercise, *Stretching for Flexibility and Health* has hopefully convinced you of the merits of doing so. Don't wait until you are in pain before doing regular exercise; usually this is costly in terms of time, treatment and management. If you exercise aerobically for 15-20 minutes, three times per week, and do a daily muscle maintenance regime, you will quickly start to tone your muscles, improve your flexibility and posture, and, best of all, feel more positive about yourself. There will always be times when you are too busy to exercise, but make sure that missing one day doesn't become an excuse for missing a month.

If you have an injury at present, which you believe prevents you from exercising, question the advice you have received, particularly if it is from a well-meaning friend. Become objective about your injury management. If rest seems unnecessarily advised, seek a second opinion. Do not give up trying to find a way, any possible way, in which you may be able to help yourself. If you are currently exercising and ignoring an injury — don't! Unfortunately, it will not "go away" without some form of intervention or treatment. Do not let the chain reaction of injury and excessive exercise damage your muscles in the long term.

Fortunately, your body really doesn't like pain — it wants to feel well and free — so what better incentive to keep your muscles healthy and fit than this?

Happy exercising, think positive and, most importantly of all, have lots of fun while staying fit!

Glossary

Actin — the thinner protein filament in the myofibrils which comprise skeletal muscle.

Active range of movement — how far an individual can move a particular part of their body, for example, lifting the arm above the head.

Adaptive shortening — the shortening that occurs over a period of time in a muscle when it is not used through its full range. For example, if the pectoral muscles are not used through their full range, adaptive shortening may occur, causing round shoulders.

Aerobic exercise — exercise that utilises oxygen from the air, to provide the energy required for exercising, for example, jogging and swimming.

Agonist — the muscle that is contracting.

Anabolic steroid — a drug taken to improve athletic performance that assists with muscle bulking. It has many negative side-effects.

Anaerobic exercise — exercise that does not depend on oxygen for its energy. There are two systems that may be used to produce the energy required for this type of exercise: the lactate and the phosphate systems.

Analgesic effect — a numbing effect exerted in an area, for example, when ice is placed on muscle tissue.

Antagonist — the muscle that relaxes and lengthens when the opposing muscle, the agonist, is contracting, the two working together to achieve balanced movement at a joint.

Artery — a strong blood vessel that is rather elastic in structure. Arteries transport oxygen-rich blood away from the heart.

Arthroscopy — a surgical procedure performed using a scope inserted via a large needle, as opposed to cutting open an area to operate. Removal of torn cartilage of the knee is commonly performed by this technique.

Ball and socket joint — a joint in which one bony surface is concave and the other convex, allowing a wide range of movement; for example, the shoulder and the hip joint.

Ballistic stretching — fast, dynamic stretching. In fitness classes, this refers to a double bounce on a muscle at the end of its range. It is potentially hazardous.

Basal metabolic rate — the rate at which the body uses energy while at rest to sustain vital bodily functions.

Bunion — a callous thickening usually found in the feet. Bunions develop where joints are being loaded abnormally.

Cardiac muscle — muscle surrounding and comprising the heart.

Cardiovascular system — the heart and the blood vessels.

Carotid arterial pulse — the pulse of the carotid artery, which can be felt at the side and slightly anterior in the neck.

Cartilage — a substance protecting the articulating surfaces at the ends of bones in joints.

Cartilaginous disc — located between each vertebra in the spine, and provides support as well as having shock-absorbing qualities.

Cell — the most basic unit of the body.

Cerebrospinal fluid — the fluid that protects and surrounds the brain and the spinal cord.

Cervical vertebrae — the seven vertebrae in the neck.

Concentric contraction — when a muscle shortens as it contracts. It is also called a positive contraction.

Connective tissue — the non-contractile white fibrous tissue that separates and supports muscles and all other visceral structures.

Counterirritant effect — occurs when another stimulus is used to override a specific pain, as when local heat rubs create a warming effect and reduce pain.

Craniosacral system — the physiological system in the human body that provides the environment in which the brain and spinal cord develop and function. Until the early 1990s this system was relatively unknown. All animals that have a brain and spinal cord (all vertebrates) possess a craniosacral system.

Dynamic stretching — stretching involves motion through a wide range at relatively fast speeds. For instance, kicking the leg high to meet an outstretched hand would be dynamic stretching of the hamstring muscle group.

Eccentric contraction — occurs when a muscle is lengthening. For example, the biceps, while lowering a weight in the hand from a flexed elbow position, are used eccentrically. It is also called a negative contraction.

Ectomorph — refers to a body type. An ectomorph is tall and thin.

Endomorph — refers to a body type. An endomorph is short and plump.

Ergometer — a piece of equipment used for fitness testing, for example, a bicycle or treadmill.

Extensor — the muscle that straightens a joint after it has been flexed. For example, the extensors of the back bring us back to the standing position when they contract, after we have bent forward touching our toes.

Fascia — a form of connective tissue that separates, supports and interconnects muscles, organs and bones. It surrounds muscles and separates them and is also found around each myofibril.

Feldenkrais method — a method of working with the body devised by Mosh Feldenkrais. Its main goal is to deprogramme poor postural and muscular habits and reprogramme new patterns by gentle awareness through movement exercises. A skilled Feldenkrais practitioner can teach the individual these movements.

Fixator — the muscle required to fix or stabilise a joint while muscles located peripherally are working more actively through their range. For example, when exercising the biceps by bending the elbows while the arms are held in horizontal abduction, the deltoid would be the fixator.

Gastrocnemius — the largest muscle below the knee, usually called the calf muscle. When it contracts, it points the foot. This is called plantaflexion.

Gastrointestinal system — all organs and parts of the system that utilises, digests and absorbs food and excretes waste products.

Gross movement — the main movement performed actively by an individual when exercising. For example, picking up an object off a table requires gross movement at the shoulder, but finer movements of the fingers.

Growth plate — occurs when new bone is laid down to permit growth in a bone, in the epiphysis (or growing end) of the bone.

Harvard step test — a very basic test that utilises a step as an ergometer to test an individual's level of fitness.

Hinge joint — any joint that permits flexion and extension but only minimal rotation. It opens and closes in a similar way to a door hinge, and occurs at the elbows, knees and toes.

Histamine — a chemical released by the body in response to pain and inflammation, and post-exercise.

Hypermobility — when an individual is overly flexible. Usually this extra flexiblity is due to extra length in the ligaments, and an increased passive range of movement is noted. It is often incorrectly labelled 'double-jointedness'.

Hypothalamic response — a response by the hypothalamus, a part of the brain. It is the means by which the body regulates and adjusts to variable temperatures.

Insertion — where a muscle attaches to bone.

Involuntary movement — when a muscle contracts suddenly without the individual thinking about contracting it. For example, an involuntary movement occurs in the arm when something very hot is touched.

Ischaemia — excessive blood pooling that occurs in muscle while exercising.

Isometric contraction — when a change in tension occurs in a muscle, but the length of the muscle stays virtually the same. For example, an isometric contraction occurs in the arm muscles during an arm wrestle.

Lactic acid — the waste product formed when glycogen (muscle energy or fuel) is only partially broken down in the absence of oxygen. Lactic acid is produced with anaerobic activity, but is removed almost entirely from the muscles and blood within 45–60 minutes after the exercise is completed. It is *not* responsible for post-exercise soreness as is commonly thought.

Ligament — a relatively inelastic fibrous band that connects bones and thus provides joint stability. Once overstrained or over-stretched, it often never returns to its original shape or strength.

Lymph nodes — small nodules found throughout the body. Accumulations are found in the armpit and groin. They are part of the lymphatic system.

Lymphatic system — the system that is primarily responsible for fighting infection in the body. It comprises lymph capillaries and lymph vessels, and these provide a pathway whereby tissue fluid is returned to the bloodstream.

Manipulation — physical techniques that influence joints or muscle with the hands. Specific joint manipulation refers to high velocity adjustments, performed by a specialised manipulative practitioner, where the patient is not able to control the movement executed on a specific joint.

Maximum heart rate — (MHR) the highest heart rate an individual will achieve. A general formula to calculate the approximate MHR is to subtract the individual's age from 220.

Mesomorph — refers to a body type. A mesomorph is of average height and muscular build.

Mobilisation — controlled graded movements, used by skilled health practitioners, to influence directly and improve the passive joint range of movement of a joint.

Multipennate — one of the muscle shapes. In this type of muscle, fibres run in many different directions. The deltoid is an example of a multipennate muscle.

Muscle — tissue that contracts to produce movement and contributes to our body shape. Muscles comprise 40 per cent of the body's mass. There are three different types of muscles: smooth, cardiac and striated. The major role of skeletal muscles is to move bones.

Musculoskeletal system — the skeleton and its associated bones, the ligaments, tendons, and the muscles.

Myofibril — the component of a muscle cell that distinguishes it from all other cells. Skeletal muscle is composed of thousands of myofibrils bound together by connective tissue and contained in a fluid called sarcoplasm.

Myosin — a myofibril contains two basic protein filaments: the thicker one is called myosin, the thinner, actin.

Nerve — part of the nervous system that carries the electrical impulses from the brain via the spinal cord. Nerves permit movement of muscle or sensation in all body parts.

Nervous system — comprises the brain, spinal cord and all nerves in the body.

Origin — the point of origin of a muscle off the bone.

Passive range of movement — how far a skilled therapist can move (i.e. mobilise or manipulate) a joint. The passive range of movement is not able to be performed by individuals themselves.

Phasic muscle — a muscle that is used (i.e. 'electrically' activated) predominately when we move.

Physical therapist — a skilled health practitioner who treats a wide range of health disorders by using physical assistance of the hands and electrotherapeutic modalities, exercise and so on.

Pivot joint — occurs where a ring of bone rotates around a bony prominence on another bone. An example is the first cervical vertebra at the base of the skull that rotates around the second cervical vertebra.

Plantafascitis — inflammation of the plantafascia, a strong fibrous strip of connective tissue that assists with the support of the arch of the foot.

PNF stretching — proprioceptive neuromuscular facilitation. One of the most effective ways to elongate a muscle, it involves contracting a muscle isometrically against an immovable object for 6–10 seconds, then relaxing the muscle before taking it into a new lengthened position, then repeating this procedure two to three times.

Podiatrist — a health practitioner who specialises in the care of feet, and who is able to assess and treat mechanical foot disorders.

Postural muscles — the muscles that are still 'electrically' active when we are standing, sitting or lying down (i.e. when we are not moving). They are also used when we move. Phasic muscles, on the other hand, are used when we move, but cease to be active when we stop.

Prime mover — the major muscle contracting in any particular movement.

Protoplasm — the jelly-like substance of the cell, where complex biochemical changes occur, forming the processes of life.

Range — how far a muscle can move a joint.

Range of movement stretching — this involves taking a muscle through the range in which it is about to be worked. For example, range of movement stretching is used in aquarobics while in the water by swinging the leg forwards and backwards from the hip to stretch the hamstrings.

Relaxin — a hormone released during pregnancy that softens the ligaments of the pelvis, hips and lower back.

Respiratory system — the lungs and air passages.

Resting heart rate — an individual's heart rate when at rest. This can be assessed by taking the pulse of a resting individual.

Skeletal muscle — also called striated muscle. It is responsible for voluntary movement of the body.

Sliding joint — a joint that moves from side to side and up and down. It can also rotate but not as freely as a ball and socket joint. Examples are the wrist and ankle joints. They are also known as ellipsoid joints.

Smooth muscle — the type of muscle found in the arteries and stomach. It is to a large extent under involuntary control.

Static stretching — occurs when a muscle is put on stretch (i.e. taken to the end of its range), held for 6–30 seconds, even longer. When the muscle is relaxed, a new length in the muscle can be achieved. This should be repeated two to three times at a minimum to be effective.

Strength training — when muscle training is done using the resistance provided by weights.

Stretch reflex — a protective reflex that prevents overstretching of a muscle. For example, if someone dozes while sitting, and the head drops forward, the stretch reflex is activated in the neck extensors, causing them to contract suddenly. This protects the neck from overstretching.

Submaximal test — a method of testing fitness where an individual is not stressed to their maximum heart rate, but figures are extrapolated from the sub-maximal test to identify how well the athlete or person will cope when they are exercising at a maximal level.

Substance P — refers to a substance produced in the body during exercise that stimulates nerve endings, causing muscle spasm, which in turn causes muscle pain.

Synergist — assists the agonist in prime movement of a body part.

Tai Chi — a series of movement and awareness exercises developed in the East. It is claimed to harmonise body forces and return them to normal.

Tendon — where a muscle approaches its attachment site with a bone, the contractile elements of that muscle end, and connective tissue known as tendons form the attachment.

Testosterone — the male hormone, though females do have some present in their bodies. It is responsible for male characteristics, such as a deepened voice and growth of hair on the chest.

Tissue — groups of cells combined together to perform a similar function.

Unipennate — the shape of a muscle where all fibres run in the same direction.

Vasoconstriction — when blood vessels (the arterioles) become smaller. This occurs when ice is placed on the body. It is under control of the sympathetic nervous system (part of the automatic nervous system).

Vasodilation — when the blood vessels (the arterioles) become larger. This occurs when heat is applied to the body. It is under the control of the parasympathetic nervous system.

Vein — a blood vessel that returns blood to the heart. It contains valves to assist the pumping of fluid up the body against gravity.

Vertebrae — the individual bones that comprise the spinal column. There are twenty-four moveable bones and seven less flexible ones.

Vertebral joints — the joints connecting the vertebrae. Each individual joint has only limited movement. However, when the vertebrae move together, the spine can bend in all directions as well as rotate.

Viscera — organs in the gastrointestinal system.

Voluntary movement — a movement performed by an individual under their own volition. For example, lifting up a cup off a table involves voluntary movement of the forearm muscles.

Index

Related Books from The Crossing Press

Sports Injuries: A Self-Help Guide
By Vivian Grisogono

This indispensable, easy-to-read, fully illustrated manual is for men and women of all ages, as well as coaches, PE teachers, and medical and paramedical practitioners interested in sports injuries.

$16.95 * Paper * ISBN 0-89594-716-1

The Healing Energy of Your Hands
By Michael Bradford

"Anyone who has come into contact with Michael Bradford knows that he channels spiritual energy with the focus of a laser beam. This energy leaps out of his book to enlighten us all."

—Lewis Walker, M.D.

$12.95 • Paper ISBN 0-89594-781-1

The Sevenfold Journey
Reclaiming Mind, Body & Spirit Through the Chakras
By Anodea Judith & Selene Vega

Combining yoga, movement, psychotherapy, and ritual, the authors weave ancient and modern wisdom into a powerful tapestry of techniques for facilitating personal growth and healing.

$18.95 * Paper * ISBN 0-89594-574-6

The Natural Remedy Book for Women
By Diane Stein

This bestseller includes information on ten different natural healing methods. Remedies from all ten methods are given for fifty common health problems.

"A must-read for women."   —*Booklist*

$16.95 * Paper * ISBN 0-89594-525-8

To receive a current catalog from The Crossing Press,
please call toll-free, 800-777-1048.
Visit our Website on the Internet at: www.crossingpress.com

Pocket Guides from The Crossing Press

Pocket Guide to Acupressure Points for Women
By Cathryn Bauer

$6.95 • Paper • ISBN 0-89594-879-6

Pocket Guide to Aromatherapy
By Kathi Keville

$6.95 • Paper • ISBN 0-89594-815-X

Pocket Guide to Ayurvedic Healing
By Candis Cantin Packard

$6.95 • Paper • ISBN 0-89594-764-1

Pocket Guide to Bach Flower Essences
By Rachelle Hasnas

$6.95 • Paper • ISBN 0-89594-865-6

Pocket Guide to Good Food
By Margaret M. Wittenberg

$6.95 • Paper • ISBN 0-89594-747-1

Pocket Herbal Reference Guide
By Debra St. Claire

$6.95 • Paper • ISBN 0-89594-568-1

Pocket Macrobiotics
By Carl Ferre

$6.95 • Paper • ISBN 0-89594-848-6

Pocket Guide to Meditation
By Alan Pritz

$6.95 • Paper • ISBN 0-89594-886-9

Pocket Guide to Naturopathic Medicine
By Judith Boice
$6.95 • Paper • ISBN 0-89594-821-4